A WOMAN'S JOURNEY FOR A LIFE DEDICATED TO GOD

Yielded

And

Submitted

A Woman's Journey for a Life

Dedicated to God

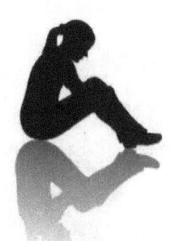

YIELDED AND SUBMITTED

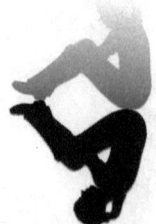

Yielded

And

Submitted

A Woman's Journey for a Life

Dedicated to God

By

Minister Onedia N. Gage

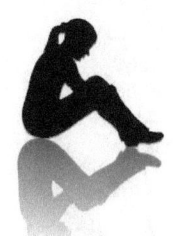

YIELDED AND SUBMITTED

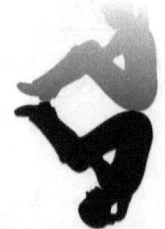

A WOMAN'S JOURNEY FOR A LIFE DEDICATED TO GOD

OTHER BOOKS BY
ONEDIA N. GAGE

As We Grow Together Daily Devotional for Expectant Couples

As We Grow Together Prayer Journal for Expectant Couples

The Blue Print: Poetry for the Soul

In Purple Ink: Poetry for the Spirit

Living An Authentic Life

Love Letters to God from a Teenage Girl

The Measure of a Woman: The Details of Her Soul

On This Journey Daily Devotional for Young People

On This Journey Prayer Journal for Young People

One Day More Than We Deserve Daily Devotional

One Day More Than We Deserve Prayer Journal

Promises, Promises

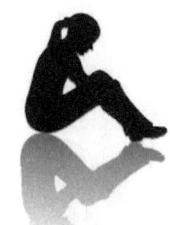

YIELDED AND SUBMITTED

Library of Congress

Yielded and Submitted
A Woman's Journey for a Life Dedicated to God

All Rights Reserved © 2012
Onedia N. Gage

No part of this of book may be reproduced or transmitted in
Any form or by any means, graphic, electronic, or mechanical,
Including photocopying, recording, taping, or by any
Information storage or retrieval system, without the
Permission in writing from the publisher.

Purple Ink, Inc. Press

For Information address:
Purple Ink, Inc
P O Box 41232
Houston, TX 77241
www.purpleink.net
www.onediagage.com

ISBN:
978-0-9801002-9-7

Printed in United States

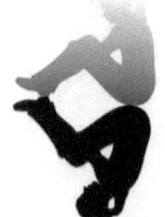

The Dedication

To the Woman who weeps in the middle of the night and who seeks God for all that He has for her but is sometimes confused and broken.

To the Woman who cries out to God but wonders if He hears her and still continues to walk in His authority.

To the Woman who wails prostrate before God in need of healing from her brokenness and a revival of her spirit.

To the Woman who wants to know how to yield unconditionally to our Father, our God, our Lord!

To the Woman He has called!

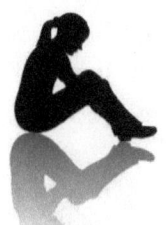

YIELDED AND SUBMITTED

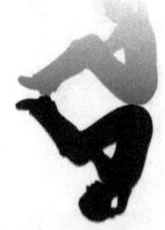

THE DEFINITIONS

Yielded [yeeld - ed] verb: to give or render as stating, rightfully owed, all required; space to give up possession of or claim or demand: to surrender or relinquish to this physical control of another; to surrender or submit (oneself) to another.

Submitted [suhb-mit] verb: to yield to governance or authority; to defer to or consent to abide by the opinion or authority of another; surrender.

To those of us who aspire to reach that level of relationship with God

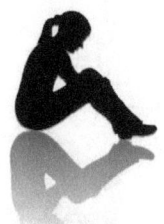

YIELDED AND SUBMITTED

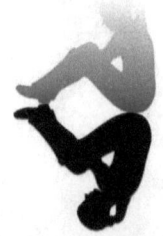

THE WORD

⁷ Submit yourselves, then, to God. Resist the devil, and he will flee from you. ⁸ Come near to God and He will come near to you. Wash your hands, you sinners, and purify your hearts, you double-minded.

¹⁰ Humble yourselves before the Lord, and He will lift you up.

James 4:7-8, 10 (NIV)

¹⁴ I praise You because I am fearfully and wonderfully made;
Your works are wonderful,
I know that full well.

Psalm 139:14 (NIV)

⁵ "Before I formed you in your mother's body I chose you.
Before you were born I set you apart to serve Me.
I appointed you to be a prophet to the nations."

Jeremiah 1:5 (NIV)

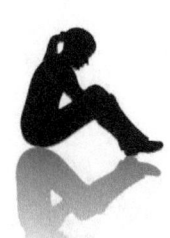

YIELDED AND SUBMITTED

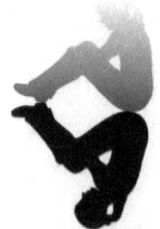

Foreword

Too often in today's society women are *forced* to yield and submit in various areas of their lives. They face yielding to less pay than men earn for doing the same job, many are asked to yield their opinions and views concerning political, social, and even religious dogmas. Women are exposed to the danger and darkness of this world; physical and emotional abuses that render them timid and fearful. Although for a good reason; they are asked in marriage vows to yield and submit to their husbands. As mothers most often mom will yield her needs to the needs and desires of her children. However, God has not given us the spirit of fear but of love, power and a sound mind. Our primary source of security is found in our relationship with our Lord and Savior Jesus Christ who is the author and finisher of our faith and the keeper of our mind body and soul.

The author guides us on a passageway to a life that reveals to us a picture of yielded and submitted life in the light of our position in Christ. I considered several definitions for the word yielded and the one that I found most appropriate for the insight presented was - "To give up one's place, as to one that is superior". When we submit our approach to life for that of God's superior plan we will discover what God's intent is for our lives.

God has created us in his own image and, God said to us through his prophet that he created us with a plan in mind - *"I know what I'm doing. I have it all planned out—plans to take care of you, not abandon you, plans to give you the future you hope for" (The Message)*. Let's be clear there is no one with breath in their body who can keep such a promise; not our mother, father, best friend, or spouse has this power, ability or love for us. So, we have nothing to lose and everything to gain in yielding and submitting our plans to the One who is truly Superior.

What does it mean to truly yield and submit? The author reveals to us images a yielded heart, mind and spirit and provides and eternal prospective of how to position ourselves in a way that we can experience the plan of God for our lives. She reminds us that God's will for us is absolute good and there is no other power in heaven or on earth that can change this. *"When I act who can reverse it"* (Isaiah 43:13b).

When we yield and submit ourselves, (our womanhood) to the sovereignty of God, the fruit of the Holy Spirit and the Light of Christ that is within every believer. The benefits and blessings of this position will render us protected from the assaults of life and any plan of the enemy to distract or derail our lives from the pathway that God has designed. She submits to us the truths of yielded and submitted life. I pray that as you read you find your strengths and weaknesses as a yielded and submitted servant of your Father and God and as a result you may discover the comfort and truth in living in the will of His way.

Minister Mattie B. Criddell

President/Founder

Oasis of Prayer Ministries

www.oasisofprayerministries.org

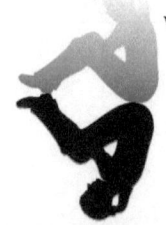

WOMAN! DEAR WOMAN OF GOD:

God has you in His hands! We need to answer Him. We are called to be yielded and submitted unto the Lord, our God. God has called us out of darkness into His marvelous light. God's calling on your life involves hard work, long days, outstanding commitment and awesome sacrifice. God's calling includes a renewed covenant with Him through His Son Jesus Christ.

We are called to yield to Him. As we enter a new life, we need to change some habits, erase excuses, eliminate drama, own our issues, address our inadequacies, and remove our doubt. Further as we enter our new life, we need to resist temptation, get out of our own way, be honest with ourselves and others, reconcile ourselves, forgive ourselves, forgive others, and learn to love ourselves.

You are reading *Yielded and Submitted: A Woman's Journey for a Life Dedicated to God* because of God's timing in your life. You are reading *Yielded and Submitted* because of God's timing in my life. *Yielded and Submitted* is testimony that God does exactly what He wants to do through us. As you read and work through *Yielded and Submitted*, consider your life with all of its success and failures. When you do, remember that those failures are designed to drive you back to God. Those success are created so that He can drive you back to Him.

Further, the testimony God develops through your life's experiences is to be shared with others. When you experienced loss and success, you help others grow when you share. Your testimony facilitates the growth of others because your testimony is a result of your personal growth. Your blessings are attached to sharing your

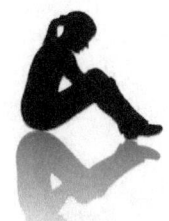

testimony. *Yielded and Submitted* is your place for change. Change that stimulates growth. Growth that produces a path back to God.

Woman, I pray that you will be blessed by *Yielded and Submitted*. Be prepared to be closer to God. Be prepared to release the issues that you have brought with you. Be prepared to be more refined and a more wonderful woman.

Be prepared to yield to God and to submit to God: to His will and His way.

In Christ's Hands,

Onedia N Gage

Onedia N. Gage

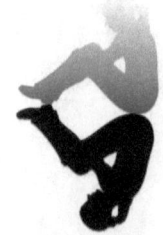

Yielded and Submitted

Introduction

' *Yielded and Submitted: A Woman's Journey for a Life Dedicated to God* was in the works for a few years. It is my personal testimony of my struggles of yielding and submitting to God. It recounts the events of the disobedience, the issues and victories. *Yielded and Submitted* demands you to address your issues, requires your accountability, and provides support throughout these pages for your experiences. Pray every step of the way; your prayers are critical. *Yielded and Submitted* requires your attention. You will be transformed by the ten topics in the text.

"The Yield Factor" designates where your life requires you to yield to God, Christ and the Holy Spirit. Yielding is required to the steps to yielding will be considered. We will also examine what the yield sign looks like. The yield sign needs to be obeyed.

"The Submission Factor" is the indicator of when we need to submit to God in a unique way. There are signals God sends calling for our submission to Him. We will experience where those areas of submission exist in our lives and those we avoid. The act of submission is an attitude. Submission is required by God so that He is able to carry forth His purposes.

"The Prayer Equation" communicates how important prayer is to our lives. The prayer commitment is one that requires our full attention. Our prayers bridge the gap and closes the areas of needs in our lives. Our prayer reconciles us to God. Prayer softens hardened hearts. Prayer provides a bridge to others we need. Prayer eliminates discomfort. Prayer addresses previously neglected areas that need to be relieved. Prayer confirms the possibility of outstanding results.

"The Faith Factor" addresses our lives which require faith. Faith is the difference in our lives. Faith is the change agent in our lives. The faith we have causes us to reconcile our life to God. Faith creates the opportunity to please God. Faith is the difference between what God wants and what God tolerates. Faith is not popular nor easy. Faith is required for the journey. God requires faith.

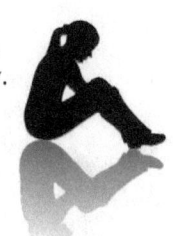

"The Fear Factor" addresses how your fear is interrupting your growth, prohibiting your relationship with God, preventing your creativity, blocking your blessings, and producing "less than" results from the blessing you are. Fear is the chemical imbalance that causes our feet to stop moving or our heart to stop desiring or our mind to stop thinking or our motivation to wane. Fear expedites failure: failure from lack of trying rather than actual attempt or effort. If you don't try, you are sure to fail.

"The Mind Factor" requires protection. Your mind is a steel trap of the assessment of your experiences, your memories of those experiences and your responses and feelings about your experience. This "steel trap" reacts to similar experiences and regulates the amount of such experiences. This "steel trap" keeps track of wrong doings and failed relationships; sometimes harboring ill feelings, holding grudges and maintaining chaos. The "steel trap" maintains the memories of excitement, when love was defined, family vacations, and other wonderful memories. Your mind needs to be protected at all costs.

"The Body Factor" also requires protection. The body cannot afford to fall into the wrong hands. The body needs to be prevented from hurt, harm, danger, ill-intent and misuse. Your body cannot be replaced. It's the only one you get. Your body requires consistent and constant protection. All visitors need to be monitored with a careful eye.

"The Lifestyle Factor" is one of excellence. In our decisions, we have to exercise excellence in our choices and discretion in those same choices. Your lifestyle affects others. We are not islands! Our choices drive our outcomes. Our choices affect an entire generation and generations to come.

"The Spirit Factor" is intentional and should be directed to God. Your spirit connects with other spirits so you have to protect how those connections are made. Your spirit will not and should not align with everyone you meet. You have to guard against unhealthy connections because that is unhealthy for your spirit and your spirit will not prosper. Your spirit is the catalyst for your growth and learning. Your spirit cannot afford to be weakened with the wrong spirits attached.

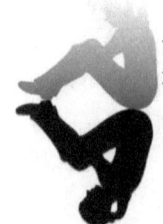

"The Self-Esteem Factor" is critically important. Both of those facilitate how you feel about yourself and consequently how you relate to others. Healthy self-esteem and a positive self-image are important. How you feel about yourself affects your professional success. Low self-esteem could potentially separate us from God.

Yielded and Submitted aligns us to God.

Yielded and Submitted drives us to God.

Yielded and Submitted develops us as better Christians and more committed to God.

Yielded and Submitted confronts those areas which interrupts your relationship with God.

Yielded and Submitted inspires you to examine your life to reconcile your dedication to God.

Yielded and Submitted requires your honest consideration of yourself and how you can become closer to the woman God wants you to be.

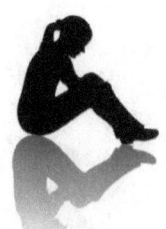

YIELDED AND SUBMITTED

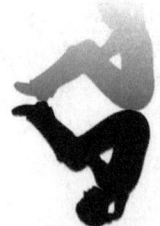

Table of Contents

Introduction	17
The Yield Factor	23
The Submission Factor	51
The Prayer Factor	55
The Faith Factor	91
The Fear Factor	119
The Mind Factor	143
The Body Factor	157
The Lifestyle Factor	177
The Spirit Factor	195
The Self-Esteem Factor	209
Yielded and Submitted: The Conclusion	217
Resources	219
Acknowledgments	233
Biography	235

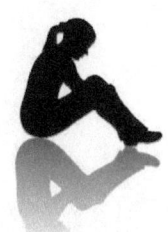

YIELDED AND SUBMITTED

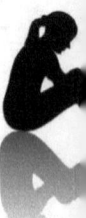

THE YIELD FACTOR

¹ Make a joyful noise unto the LORD, all ye lands.

² Serve the LORD with gladness: come before his presence with singing.

³ Know ye that the LORD he is God: it is he that hath made us, and not we ourselves; we are his people, and the sheep of his pasture.

⁴ Enter into his gates with thanksgiving, and into his courts with praise: be thankful unto him, and bless his name.

⁵ For the LORD is good; his mercy is everlasting; and his truth endureth to all generations.

Psalm 100
King James Version (KJV)

Yield is defined as to give up, as to superior power or authority according to dictionary.com. Yield is used as a verb, which means to yield requires action. As a driver in the driving world, to yield is at least a pause for the oncoming traffic to clear past. Sometimes that yield sign requires a longer pause—a complete stop. Both of those activities are for our safety. A spiritual yield is to wait on God, Christ or/and the Holy Spirit for direction(s). To yield to God means that you are waiting on His direction to go forward. You are in a prayerful, meditative state, so you can hear from God about the direction you need to take to be aligned with God's will.

When we consider yield, to whom do we yield, we yield to God, Jesus and the Holy Spirit and what He has called us to do so. What does it mean to yield to God? Yielding to God means that we hand over all of who we are back to our Creator. Each and every detail

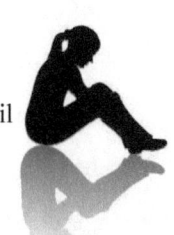

of who we are is to be yielded to God. He created each of those details of who we are and those details belong to God and they are designed to serve Him.

Yield means that I will give over my thoughts to God. My thoughts should do the following: 1) bring glory to God, 2) consider what God wants for my life, and, 3) serve others because I think of what God wants for me to do for others.

Yield means I will give my heart to God. My heart and by extension the things I am passionate about also should be focused on God and those things which bring God glory.

When we yield to God, Jesus and the Holy Spirit, great events happen. Let's not get caught up with the material and tangible or people beings. I refer to great events such as a journey back to God because you have some distance between you and Christ. When we yield to Him, He is able to create within us a clean heart, forgive us our sins, heal us from our afflictions, prosper our souls, hear us when we pray and answers our prayers.

As we come to define and redefine yield as relates to God, we need to consider that we yield our hearts, minds, energy and spirit to God.

Who do we yield to? We yield to a lot of elements and persons and situations. We are supposed to yield to God, Christ and the Holy Spirit. Yielding is not easy. God requires us to yield to Him. Yielding is an act of submission and total surrender to God because of respect.

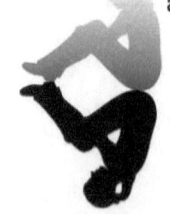

When we consider the Scripture reference, which opened our chapter, we have to consider the elements of those verses which speak to yielding to God. In order to serve the Lord with gladness and come before His presence with singing, you have to yield to God. Yielding is void of pride. As the sheep, we are to yield to the Shepherd. As we have defined the word yield, yield involves total surrender. When we consider how we are told to come before the Lord that activity is an act of yielding. Our very posture communicates a yielded spirit. This posture pleases God and reminds Him that we are aware of how our posture gives Him glory.

Who Do We Yield To

The first persons we yield to are our God, Jesus Christ, and the Holy Spirit. We yield to them individually and collectively. God is the Creator of me and everything and everyone. We yield to God because He is Creator. Jesus Christ deserves our yielding because He died for our sins. God plans for us. He created us with that purpose in mind. He has a destiny for us (Jeremiah 29:11). God knows us and we don't know all of what God will do in our lives. We yield because He is worthy of our yielding. He deserves our attention. He gives us everything we need spiritually, physically, emotionally and physiologically. He creates within us the desires we have. He gives us our victories. He disciplines us when we are wrong. He gives us what He desires for us to do. God gives us the ability to dream. He gifted us with Jesus Christ, His only son. He then gifted us with the Holy Spirit. He left us with an incomprehensible love, which overwhelms us when we try to share its power with others. His love is the best thing that ever happened to us. His forgiveness is the second best gift He ever gives us. We yield to God first and most often.

We yield to Jesus Christ, our Lord and Savior. First, of all, Jesus is the son of God who was born of a virgin, Mary and her husband, in a manger at night in "winter." To Him, we yield. Jesus is the sacrifice for my unborn sins. Jesus Christ lived sin free for 33 years and His life ended in a tragically short, while God—timed crucifixion. Jesus taught us to pray. Jesus fed us. Jesus teaches. Jesus preaches. Jesus reminds us that He loves us when our fear is strongest. Jesus reminds us that He loves through our storms. Jesus reminds us that He loves us because of our growth, whether willingly or unwillingly. Jesus keeps us from falling, failing and faltering. Jesus serves as an example of how to obey God, walk away from sin, avoid temptation and love the least of us. Jesus teaches us to be angry and still not sin! Keeping up with Jesus is a task which is not something that can be done easily but following His instructions can be done. Jesus makes one ask how can I stop sinning. Jesus healed the brokenhearted, the ill and the lonely. Jesus hung out with sinners and shared His love unselfishly. Jesus shares His heart unselfishly.

Keep in mind that we use the present tense to share what Jesus did during His life because although His physical life is over, the examples are alive, present, and completely applicable. Jesus serves others the way He should be served. Jesus saves lives: from four days of death to walking around dead while appearing alive. Jesus believes in us basically because we don't call forward the faith we were born with. Jesus comforts us when we are burdened and weary and require rest. Jesus considers us His friends. Friends require a special

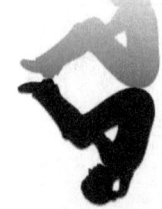

relationship. Friends seek to understand the other friend to grow closer to one another. Jesus cares about my soul and my heart and my spirit. Jesus reminds us that "they" persecuted Him first. Jesus humbled Himself to be baptized by the one who paved the way. Jesus washes our feet in an effort to share what we should do for others. Jesus blesses us for just trying to love Him; even when we are disobedient. We yield to Jesus Christ!

We yield to the Holy Spirit. The Holy Spirit is gifted to us by Jesus Christ to intercede for us. The Holy Spirit intercedes when we don't know what to pray for. The Holy Spirit intercedes for us when we don't know what to pray for with groans that God understands for our good. The Holy Spirit fuels our understanding of God. The Holy Spirit facilitates the Spirit of discernment which He shares with us so that we can connect to the will of God. The Holy Spirit comforts us when we are in pain, despair, hurt, morally bankrupt or socially marginalized. The Holy Spirit creates in us a hungry soul for God. The Holy Spirit shares our hurt with compassionate behavior and an understanding attitude. The Holy Spirit offers direction and delivers shelter. The Holy Spirit protects with the dedication of Jesus. The Holy Spirit steers with the guidance of God. The Holy Spirit recognizes our fervor and zeal. The Holy Spirit dwells within us. The Holy Spirit controls our knowledge of God. The Holy Spirit defies the ordinary, the impossible, the normal and the expected. The Holy Spirit pleads for us with God. The Holy Spirit is responsible for the power that is within us to understand the love of God (Ephesians 3:14-21). The Holy Spirit presents us with particular power which fuels the work to which we are assigned. The Holy Spirit bridges the gap in our relationship with God and Christ. The Holy Spirit assists us with what God wants us to know through either God or Jesus. The Holy Spirit redeems us.

We yield to God, Jesus Christ and the Holy Spirit. We yield to the directions, instructions, love, discipline, and discernment. We yield our pride, attitudes, issues and sins to God, Jesus and the Holy Spirit.

When We Yield to God, Jesus Christ and the Holy Spirit

We need to yield daily! How difficult is it to yield to God, Jesus Christ, and the Holy Spirit? The difficult part of yielding is knowing to yield, knowing when to yield, knowing why to yield, and knowing to share and how to share the results of that yielding.

Luke 9:23 reads: "Then He said to them all: "Whoever wants to be My disciple must deny themselves and take up their cross daily and follow Me.""

In order to do that, yielding is required. You cannot follow Christ without yielding to God. Yielding daily is an interesting proposition—one requiring sacrifice and focus, commitment and perseverance.

Yielding is similar and synonymous to surrender. Give it all over to God. "It" is All of you. I preached a sermon entitled "I Am All In." God requires all of us given to Him. In this sermon, I explain a poker strategy labeled "I'm all in." This move is one where with complete faith in her cards, the player places all of her money in the table's center and declares, "I'm all in." This move signifies to the other players that she is serious about her cards. She is willing to give

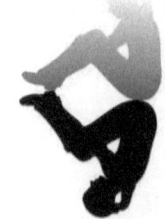

all that she has. The other players recognize her sincerity and they have to meet her efforts or they need to fold or quit. This acknowledgement of her cards is the most sacrificial move she can make. This is what yielding looks like to God.

When we yield, we increase our relationship with the Trinity. The total surrender to God, Holy Spirit and Jesus Christ places us in the best possible position to hear from God or Jesus or the Holy Spirit. The answers to our questions, fears, worries, and the anxieties rest with our yielding. When we do not yield, we distance ourselves from these possibilities. When we yield, we open ourselves up to God's fullness. We completely open ourselves to Him and His undeserved mercy, favor and grace.

When we yield, we express our love to God, Jesus and the Holy Spirit.

On our way back to God, our yielding communicates that we recognize His sovereignty. God's mercy covers us from our own self.

What Do We Yield To

As a woman, Christian, and human, I yield to things and stuff which cause me to distance myself from God. That distance determined by sin is how I got away from God anyway. We move away from God, God does not move away. I have "yielded" to some, a bunch of ridiculous stuff—sins which really cause me to question my actual consciousness.

YIELDED AND SUBMITTED

I have subjected myself to some demeaning events which I may never share with another human being. This is also not the time to compare sins. What we have done is not important—it is all called sin. All sins are EQUAL. Just because I will not do what you have done does not make me better. We are not authorized to judge each other's sins. Likewise, we cannot justify our own.

The most important thing that we all can do is to ask God forgiveness and TRUST He has forgiven and LEAVE it there! The sin which we perpetually commit is that we ask forgiveness but we keep beating ourselves up for what we have done.

The yielding we do to God keeps us from sinning. There is a choice to be made: God versus sin. When I choose God, I reject sin. I need to work on consistently choosing God and rejecting sin. Paul tells us in Romans 7 that "For I have the desire to do what is good, but I cannot carry it out. For I do not do the good I want to do, but the evil I do not want to do—this I keep on doing."

As we consider "what" we actually yield to, I sincerely implore that we examine the specific sins which cause us the greatest distance with God. We have to poise ourselves with God to pray past those issues and temptations. God states He provides us an escape from the sin which tempts us (1 Corinthians 10:13). Do we always recognize the escape route? Do we always use the escape route?

God wants NO DISTANCE between us and Him. He wants us to rest in HIS bosom. Remain in the safety of His hands. Rely on His voice for wisdom. Request His forgiveness when we stray from His directions. He would like us to research His words. Recall His works.

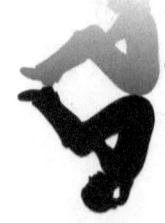

THE YIELD FACTOR

Remember His discipline. Remove our fears. Relinquish our pride. Repeat our walk of faith. Remind ourselves of His love. Return to His shelter, the safety only He can provide. When we yield to God and let Him give us what we need, then we reaffirm His power. He shares this power which is at work within us. Resort to His image, the one He used to make us. The image we consistently rearrange based on what others say, do, feel and criticize. Revive the love we reject daily because we do not understand how to relax in His profound love. If we understood His love and could be loved the way He defined us, then we could close the gap between God and us.

We yield so that He can remind us that He is holding us close to Him.

We yield to close that gap between God and us.

Why Do We Yield

I question God often because I am a precocious and inquisitive child but I try to avoid asking why. That is my personal boundary with God. In my early Christian walk, I have boldly, almost disrespectfully, asked God why about many issues. But my favorite question was 'why me God?' God's answer: "Why not you, Onedia?" God extended His answer on several occasions and His answer included: "Because I am Sovereign, I am your God, your Provider, your Comforter. I have a plan for you and this is part of it. I have provided you peace of mind. I gave you that heart so you have to love others. I sustain you when the persons I assigned to you to love, hurt you. I hold you when you are lonely. I hug you when you are about to embarrass Me at the retail counter. I dry your tears because I tell you I love you and My love is

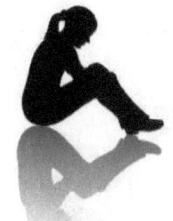

comprehensively enough. I keep your past out of your face. I forgive you when you ask—others don't forgive you and sometimes you regard them higher. So Onedia, My question is why not you? I know your FULL potential. I love you unconditionally!"

I usually cry as a result of that encounter!

We yield because He loves us. When we love Him back that only elevates the relationship. We yield because we won't error when we do so. Yielding is a respect factor. Between love and respect, yielding will come easily. Love causes the yielding to happen because of your relationship. Relationships require some things to happen. Respect causes behavior to salvage itself. Because of respect of another we may treat them differently than others. We are aware that we treat people differently because of the love, respect, and relationship we have. As it is with God, the closer we grow to Him, the more committed we are to yield.

We yield because we need God and His order for our steps His plans and His redemption. We need God, Jesus and the Holy Spirit. We are His tools, His instruments, His elements—which He uses in the lives of others to do the work He has already planned for each of us. We cannot do His work or serve His purpose if we do not yield.

How Do We Yield

We yield through our behavior, particularly our sin, or lack thereof. There is total surrender in the ability to yield. To yield is to SUBMIT to God and His will. To yield is the clause we use when we tell God that we are ready to do whatever He wants us to do. To yield is

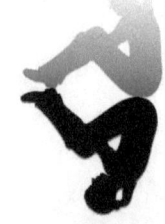

to check our behavior, attitude and our selfishness. To yield is to give all of that over to God so that He can repair us and make us useful for God's people and His work. To yield is confessing our sins to God and knowing that our confession restores us to wholeness with God.

We yield when we love others. We yield when we serve others. We yield when we seek God. We yield when we study God's word. We yield when we pray regularly and diligently. We yield when we intercede on behalf of others by request or Spirit led.

Yielding maybe difficult if we are out of God's will. In order to return to God's will, we would need to avoid sin. Yielding means we acknowledge that need to avoid sin. Yielding means recognizing that God is our Rock and Redeemer. Yielding introduces obedience at a sacrificial level. Yielding is Luke 9:23—denying self daily. Yielding includes sharing with God that you need His leadership.

Yielding remains calm and focused on His word.

OUR YIELDED EXAMPLES

When we consider biblical persons who have yielded unto God and submitted to His will, there are a few immediate names which present themselves. They will be in three groups: those who were willing to yield, those who were initially unwilling to yield, and those who were yielded from birth. In the next few pages we will discuss our examples: Hagar, Elizabeth, Naomi, Ruth, the woman with the issue of blood, Paul, Mary, David and John the Baptist. They had to yield through their circumstances. They learned the value of yielding.

YIELDED AND SUBMITTED

Just a Servant (Genesis 16)

The story of Hagar is less than deserved. Hagar is offered to Abraham because Sarah wanted a child badly and had become impatient with God. Sarah did not anticipate Abraham's new attitude toward Hagar. To them was born Ishmael. Sarah sends Hagar away. Abraham doesn't know what to do and seeks God. God assures Abraham that He will provide for Hagar and Ishmael, to remain with Sarah and remain faithful. Abraham meekly obeyed. Ishmael was given the land that God promised. Hagar was protected and provided for and cast away but still loved. Hagar had God. She was also elevated due to her obedience and attitude about the issues she faced. Hagar was a maid servant. Hagar became a mother and one whose child God would raise to a high position because of his lineage, affording her the privileges of that same inheritance. Hagar could have chosen several different actions but she did just as God told her.

Old Yet Willing (Luke 1:5-25, 39-45)

Elizabeth was well up in years, however we do not know how old that is, and was barren. She and her husband were a content couple, doing what God said until the angel visited with Zechariah to share with him that Elizabeth would have a child. Elizabeth believed and was calm and faithful! Zechariah was silent until the birth of John the Baptist due to disbelief, while Elizabeth marveled at God's decision and faithfulness.

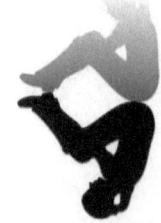

Further, Elizabeth is Mary's cousin. Mary visits to share her news only to discover Elizabeth's fortune. At which time, these women understand completely the weight they actually carry.

THE YIELD FACTOR

Elizabeth counseled Mary about the pregnancy and whatever else Mary wanted to share. They use this time to commune with each other as well as worship God. In this meeting is when John the Baptist is able to acknowledge Jesus while still in the womb. Elizabeth says that he leapt inside. We learn later that he already recognized Jesus as the Christ and Savior. Essentially they were doing what God called them to do and they did it willingly.

Their unique circumstances brought them together with faith and drawing them still closer to God. God used these two yielded, related women to fulfill an awesome prophecy.

At the Top of a Strong Tree (Ruth)

Naomi and Ruth are always examples of who God uses. Yielding is all about attitude and willingness. Naomi was suffering from an unloved state. She could not 'see' God's hand on her life because of her multiple loses within her family. Ruth would not leave her. The family structure somewhat different than now. There was a lineage order which was respected and followed very carefully and closely.

Naomi's wisdom suggested that Ruth find a safe place to work for food and protection. Naomi had a relative, Boaz, but it did not seem proper to seek him out directly. However, Ruth meets Boaz because of her work ethic. The scripture states that he inquires about her to the lead attendant. Boaz takes immediate interest by assuring that she is not touched. In that regard, Boaz has labeled her as his in that he is willing openly to protect her from others while she is not legally his wife.

YIELDED AND SUBMITTED

Ruth makes a responsive move which involved discretion and poise. She confirms her interest which makes him move forward with the pursuit of her. There are two steps Boaz had to take in the community: waiting on another relative who has first right of refusal and a meeting with the elders to confirm the commitment. The elder concedes to Boaz the property of Naomi is inclusive of Ruth being his wife.

Ruth did two things: persistence to stay with Naomi although she was not obligated to do so and she listened to her mother-in-law. She yielded to a larger plan and community because she was meek, humbled and most importantly, yielded to God.

As a result, she wed Boaz. The Lord was gracious and "enabled her to conceive" a son. The Lord's favor is comprehensive based on the fact that Boaz and Ruth are the great-grandparents of David, King David, who was highly favored by God. This is a result of yielding to God.

Naomi had to renew her hope and faith. Naomi was restored and respected in her community. She had learned much from the daughter-in-law who stayed. Naomi is a major example of persistence when giving up is the first thought. Ruth loved Naomi unconditionally. Naomi wasn't ready for that initially and really did not know how to manage Ruth's love. She finally yielded and life evolved. She also realized that God's hand and favor had never left her.

For Twelve Years (Luke 8:43-48)

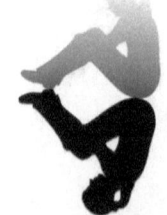

THE YIELD FACTOR

Yielding is never so evident as with the woman with the issue of blood. In that time this woman, who will call Woman for this illustration, was not supposed to be in the general population. Three things happen to this woman: (1) She has tried everyone but Jesus; (2) She found out about Jesus; and, (3) She sought Jesus with all that she had. The Woman realized that ONLY JESUS could heal her and her situation. That's yielding to Jesus. She recognized that her strength did not heal her. Her healing was not in her power. Her surrender to God, and Jesus did heal her!

The Woman took a risk on faith that Jesus would heal so she pushed through the crowd, where she wasn't supposed to be, to get to Jesus, who she wasn't supposed to touch, to have healing she had just about given up on experiencing, and she was healed IMMEDIATELY. She presses through the crowd and gets past security—the Twelve—to Jesus. She intended to go unnoticed. She touched Jesus and was IMMEDIATELY healed. While she quietly rejoiced, she did not know how exactly sensitive Jesus was to His own power. She didn't count on Him stopping to seek her. She thought He would just think it was the crowd as the disciples said. Jesus persisted to see who touched Him. He knew that power "left" Him to heal someone and He wanted to know who it was. He asked to complete the healing. He already knew. He wanted to affirm her in front of others.

Finally, she renewed her courage and stepped forward to admit to Jesus that she was the one. Jesus as usual surprised her and the Twelve. He spoke directly to her saying, "Daughter, your faith has healed you. Go in peace." (Luke 8:48).

This encounter raised several questions: (1) Are we in position to yield to Jesus? (2) Are we willing to risk all that we are and have to seek Jesus for our needs and desires? (3) Are we sure that we understand His true level of sensitivity for us and our pains and victories? (4) Are we steady enough to keep the prescribed course Jesus has planned for your no matter how hard the path? (5) Are we bold enough to say, Jesus it is me who seeks You for my needs and forgiveness and love? (6) Are we able to share what God has done for us so others will know that God is real and invite others to meet God for themselves? (7) Have we placed all of our FAITH in Him for all we are, ask, need and wish? If not, when will we? (8) When He makes us whole, will we share our testimony with a Jesus—ordained transparency? (9) When He makes us complete, will we praise and worship Him in the manner in which He deserves? (10) As we yield, may we relax our excuses and obstacles so that we can serve God as He gifted, called and created us to serve Him?

The Woman teaches how to recognize the worth of Christ, the value of seeking Christ, how to reject the judgment of others and how to PRESS through to meet God. She yielded to the power of God and His love! That power is powerful enough to move our obstacles and carry all of our burdens!

ALMOST DID NOT YIELD

Those examples are of those who were in a willing posture to yield. Our next examples are those who were the most unlikely to EVER yield: Paul/Saul, the woman at the well, and Peter. Let's visit with them.

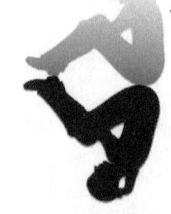

Oh Ye of Little Faith (Matthew 14:22—36)

Peter seemed willing but often found himself in a quandary for what to do. Peter has been selected to follow Christ and to train others to do the same. Within that training to follow Christ, he seems willing as long as he has the opportunity to question and challenge Christ about His decisions, methods, and activities. Peter positions himself to question whatever Christ does. Peter was the first disciple selected. As they traveled, Peter witnessed Jesus heal many, even his own mother-in-law in his home. Even with ALL of that, Peter asks the big question, poses the big challenge: "If it is You, Jesus, then call me out to You!" Matthew 14:28. Peter tells Jesus to invite him to walk on water. As if ALL of the other events were not enough to prove what He can and will do. Peter is the same one who tell Christ that people are crowding around Him and there was no possible way to know who touched Him but Jesus insisted that He needed to find who it was. Peter continues down this path with the requests for explanations. Then there was the denial of Jesus.

Again we are considering the ability and willingness to yield. Peter is in the perfect position to yield to Christ. Peter yields sparingly or rather without prime regard for the image it gives Christ that His first disciple is the worst in the simple belief in Jesus just because of what Peter has witnessed. Peter SAW it ALL!! Multiple times Peter still questioned Christ, lacked faith at times, and denied Jesus three times just as Jesus predicted! Peter had the benefit of walking with Jesus, having unlimited access to Him and didn't take full advantage. Instead some of the questions Peter ask such as, "Lord, are you telling this parable to us, or to everyone?" Gage's response is, "Peter, does it

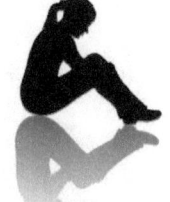

matter?" Peter should have taken the lesson as it was presented. Peter is not alone in this. We get off task so easily. Jesus is trying to teach us something valuable each time He walks, talks, and even breathes. Why would Peter show his cluelessness in this manner? Peter's wisdom should be more evident than this.

There are times when Jesus has to chastise and challenge us into a yielding spirit. Sometimes we act just like Peter. This is not a yielded spirit. Jesus spends time with us in a similar manner. Jesus has to "convince" us that yielding is important, that He is worthy and He is qualified.

Eventually Peter yields and submits to Christ in a manner which demonstrates that he believes that yielding is valuable. Peter pleases Christ with his new attitude which is the result of Christian maturity.

The Woman at the Well (John 4:1—26)

The woman at the well was offered an opportunity to yield and she also declined. This speaks volumes about how we respond when Christ addresses us. She immediately declines that Jesus is correct about His observations. He shares the details of her life with her. She declines the entire dialogue. When she finds out that she speaking with Jesus, she really doesn't change her defensive posture.

We cannot be yielded if we are defensively postured. We have to be humbly postured when we seek Him, when we serve Him, and when we sin. Defending our choices, which are consequently our sins in an unyielding attitude and posture, displeases and offends God.

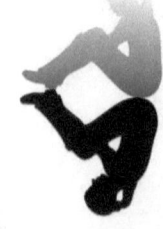

THE YIELD FACTOR

The other lesson she teaches us is that as we approach Christ that we are honest with God about our sins and our wrongdoings.

The well woman didn't want to admit that she had sinned but Jesus did not pose a question to which He did not know the answer. Jesus asked her to see if she would be truthful rather than for the actual answer, which He already knew. Jesus wants that for us and in order to be yielded we have to be honest and transparent. Often we hold back from Christ what we should be willing to openly confess as we want the desires of our heart but neglect the part about delighting ourselves in Christ. When we "delight" ourselves, we are yielded in Christ in a unique manner. We are poised to address Jesus with the person we have chosen to be. We are already far away from the factory settings with which we are born.

She later responded as a yielded woman truly grateful to have been forgiven by Jesus. He has permitted her to go forward with a better outlook on life and self-worth, and that life allowed for her to do the work He assigned. This is what He wants for us as well. Our daily questions should be how can I yield better to Jesus? What can I remove to better yield to God? Once these and other similar questions are answered then we can better address our fleshly desires, deny ourselves and follow Him (Luke 9:23) and yield to God as He requires.

With a Transformation and Transfiguration (Acts 9)

Paul is the epitome of my new self. Saul was OUTSPOKEN against Christ. Saul was a killer and an all around sinner. Does Saul resemble anyone you know? Yes, of course, Saul is just like each of us before we met, and became intimate with Christ. Saul had no intention

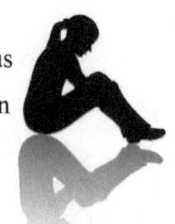

to LOVE Christ or do anything that was Christ-like. Saul was a SINNER. Like all of us who believe we are self-made. In this state, we are living recklessly and foolishly. Our behavior sends God a message that we are rebellious and disrespectful. We tell God that we do not understand what He does and who He is.

As we follow the life of Saul, he continues to speak out against the word of God. Not only does Saul not understand why he is alive, Saul does not understand that we are alive so that God can use us. Saul thinks that he is invincible. Acts 9:1 reads, "Meanwhile, Saul was still breathing our murderous threats against the Lord's disciples." Verse 3, Acts 9 states that there was a light from heaven which surrounded him. In verse 4, Jesus speaks to Saul asking 'why do you persecute Me.' Saul's weak reply starts the conversion Jesus had planned. Saul's speechlessness then prompted Jesus continued to tell Saul what to do. Saul has now surrendered. This event prompted a yielding that Saul had not anticipated.

Jesus knew that in order to use Saul, He needed to do something significant. This immediate and invasive approach was the ONLY way to get Saul's attention. Some of us have BIG stories like this: the manner by which God got our attention was so great that we are within His will immediately. For some of us we need to have the ability to negotiate or come on our own to Christ eliminated TOTALLY. Some of us have to be without choices in order to choose CHRIST!

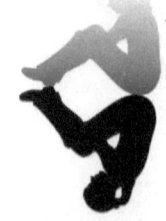

Saul did not have any processing time. There was not 'Jesus-wait-a-minute-I'll-be-right-there' speech that many of our testimonies start with. There was not 'the-Lord-let-me-get-it-straight-then-I'll-do-everything-You-want' discussion. Jesus addressed Saul, called him into service, sent Ananias, a disciple, to restore his sight, told Ananias what Saul's job was and immediately put His will in motion. Jesus converted Saul from an enemy of the gospel to the gospel's greatest preacher in a matter of hours. Acts 9, verse 20 reads: "At once he began to preach in the synagogues that Jesus is the Son of God." Jesus does not tarry when He wants us or when He is ready for us to do His work, be within His will and follow Him. Further, Jesus does not wait on us to decide to follow Him. Saul had NO intentions but Jesus' plan prevailed and will prevail all the time. God said that His word will not return void.

Verse 21 is the verse that should arrest our attention. [21]All those who heard him were astonished and asked, "Isn't he the man who raised havoc in Jerusalem among those who call on this name? And hasn't he come here to take them as prisoners to the chief priests?" Acts 9:21. Is that not how we sound when we doubt those called by God who have previously sinned? Is that what we do? We question how God could call someone like Saul to teach about Jesus. We compare our sins to someone like Saul and say with a judgmental tone that God did not choose someone worthy of who we would call. We cannot compare our sins to that of others. ALL sins are equal. Jesus uses Saul to send us a well-constructed message that He can use whoever He wants to do whatever He wants. This includes us.

Jesus also uses who will yield. Jesus is not interested in our excuses or our agendas or our timeframes for when it is convenient to yield to Him. You know the ones I referred to earlier, in addition to the talk of self-doubt which is when we announce we are unworthy to serve God. This very example serves as notice of the fact that because we are unworthy yet willing to yield thus serve Him, He will restore us to Him so that we will be effective in our calling. It is pure speculation on the author's behalf to believe Jesus selected Saul to preach after ALL the persecution of Jesus' name because Jesus trusted that Saul would preach an UNCOMPROMISED gospel. Based on Saul's previous behavior, Jesus knew the weight of the message that Saul would present would be effective to lead the lost to Christ. Saul had been effective with creating doubt, instilling fear and generally threatening those who might believe, so he was seen with GREAT potential for someone who would do a GREAT job for God as he had attempted to do against God.

Consider the question Jesus poses: why do you persecute me. As a student of the text, I wonder if I am correct in concluding that Jesus' tone indicates that Saul does not know Him well enough to persecute. Saul's answer to the question: 'Who are You, Lord?' is an indicator that my conclusion is correct. Just as anyone does, we will say ANYTHING about someone whom we do not know or have deep enough relationship. However, when we have a relationship, we protect that person. We say only GREAT things to that person and about that person.

Jesus trusted Saul to do His will. The Bible says that God knew us before we were formed in our mother's womb (Jeremiah 1:5). This word applies to the people in the Bible as well. Jesus knew that Saul would behave this way until Saul was formally introduced to Jesus. As we read on in Acts, Saul does not ask Jesus anything else. Saul does not disobey the directions. Saul goes forward with Jesus' instructions and does so immediately. We cannot say that about

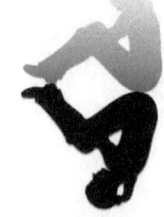

THE YIELD FACTOR

ourselves. Saul behaved and was yielded to Jesus. We need a warning, an email, a text message, a memo, several confirmations and we would like Jesus to ask for our permission to be used by Him, when He created us and He needs to make an appointment to ask for our consent! WE need to YIELD! Until we yield, we will have trouble with receiving our assignments.

Saul went on to preach the gospel, was well received by the audiences and because of the messages, many were committed to Christ. Eventually Saul became Paul. Paul continued ministering throughout the land. Paul certainly asserted himself as a Christian yielded to God, Jesus and the Holy Spirit.

YIELDED FROM BIRTH

This next group is those who were yielded from birth: Mary, John the Baptist, and David.

A Man After God's Own Heart (1 Samuel 16:11-12)

David was appointed King at 12 years old. David was chosen by God to serve as King after Saul (not the same Saul in the New Testament). David served with Saul. During this time, David had to remain humble and focused on God's calling. David has done incredible work for God. David yielded to God immediately and remained yielded to God. David was labeled as the man after God's own heart. David communed with God so that he could hear from God. David shows us how to praise, worship, and love God. David teaches how to grieve, celebrate, and repent, all in one afternoon. David

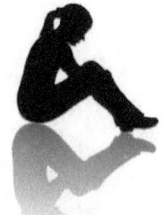

touched many lives and shared with many the love of God. David worked hard to live a life God would be proud of because of his calling.

God invested heavily in David. David is the midpoint of well-documented, highly-favored lineage. Ruth is his great-grandmother. Jesus is his descendant fourteen generations away. David had tremendous faith: A faith pleasing to God.

David made a few notable errors however, because of God's grace and mercy, God restored David to Himself. David demonstrates yielded to God through mind, body, soul and spirit.

Because of a Virgin (Luke 1:26-38, 46-56)

Mary was a teenager who was selected to carry Jesus Christ, our Savior, for nine months as a virgin. Mary was born a yielded spirit. The argument would clearly be how does one confidently make such an assumption. Mary was a virgin and promised to Joseph. Mary was selected above all other eligible women. Mary carried the baby for nine months. Mary consented with her heart to God and her body through purity. Mary was responsive to God when the angel visited her about the calling on her life.

Not just anyone can carry our Savior. I would feel unworthy. Although we may all feel unworthy, we are actually unworthy. Mary may have been unworthy but Mary was yielded.

In Mary's testimony, God believed she would endure and she did. He knew she could remain pure. What can God trust us with? Mary made a sacrificial offering with her body to God and was greatly

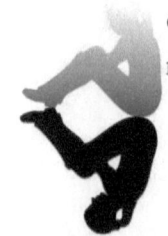

THE YIELD FACTOR

rewarded for yielding to God. She did not ask "Why me?" She did not even understand what this meant in total.

Are we willing to be totally sacrificed for the glory of God? Could He have chosen one of us? Can He choose one of us? Can we live a life worthy of being chosen for the absolute glory of God?

When I witness the testimonies of other women, I consider the profound relationship they must have with God.

Mary's story does not end there. Mary goes on to be married to Joseph, have other children, and to worship her Son, The Son of God. Mary lived past the looks and the sneers of those He could not choose to be the transportation for their Savior. My favorite Mary story is when she is rubbing Jesus' feet with her hair. Her sister, Martha, exclaims to Jesus to make her help in the kitchen. Jesus tells Martha that Mary is doing what is important: worshipping her Lord while He is physically present. This lesson transcends Martha's immediate comprehension.

When we consider what we give God of us, is that enough? Are we really yielded to God so we can be used in a GREAT way? Most of us are limited for use because of attitude and limitations we place in God's way. Mary denied herself and ignored the world to serve God. Mary never asked what will Joseph think or will Joseph leave me. An amazing servant!

Recognized While In the Womb (Luke 1:44, 57-66; John 1:19-28)

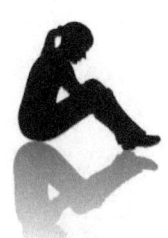

John the Baptist was responding to Jesus before their births! At their meeting while in the womb, John the Baptist leapt inside Elizabeth. That is the definition of yielded even before birth. John knew his role upon arrival. There was no ambiguity and he was trusted to carry out his calling.

John was humble enough to share with those who were assigned to him who Jesus was. John was asked several times if he was the Messiah. He humbly and promptly said no. He went on to share that he was unworthy to tie the sandals of the One who was to come, yet he baptized Jesus!

God assigned John to lead the way for Jesus. John did exactly what God designed for him. John the Baptist was one authentic Christian. John was not a disciple. Initially this perplexed me. I did not understand why he was not a disciple. Rather he prepared the way for the disciples. John was more mature than the disciples regarding the knowledge of Jesus so he would not be a match what the disciples are trying to become equipped to do. John died while serving Jesus and preaching so that others could love our Christ.

John defines yielded.

Rewards of Yielding

Based on our study of the ten yielded examples, we know that there are God—sized and ordained rewards for yielding to God, Jesus Christ and the Holy Spirit.

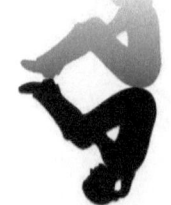

The rewards of yielding are:

THE YIELD FACTOR

1. Closer relationship with God, Christ and the Holy Spirit.
2. Your testimony is stronger.
3. You are reaping the benefit of the perseverance to submit to God's will.
4. Obedience to God which communicates our love to God.
5. An attitude change for you based on understanding the difference in God's will when we are committed to God rather than just involved with God. There's a HUGE difference between commitment and involvement.
6. Your testimony will grow others in Christ.
7. This new and renewed relationship will cause you to live consistently for Christ.
8. Your faith has made you a more complete Christian.
9. You earned God's favor because His trust in you has been proven.
10. You have the confidence to encourage others to follow Christ more closely.

Consider how God wants us to yield, individually and collectively. In order for Him to be completely glorified, we have to yield. TOTALLY. We cannot hold anything back nor can we think that the portion of ourselves which we retain is hidden from God. Do not be mistaken: we cannot withhold anything from God without His consent.

Take careful inventory about what you need to do so that you can be yielded to God.

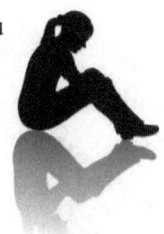

YIELDED AND SUBMITTED

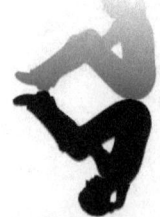

THE SUBMISSION FACTOR

"If you love Me, keep My commands."

John 14:15
New International Version (NIV)

⁷Serve wholeheartedly, as if you were serving the Lord, not people, ⁸because you know that the Lord will reward each one for whatever good they do, whether they are slave or free.

Ephesians 6:7-8
New International Version (NIV)

Jesus replied: "Love the Lord your God with all your heart and with all your soul and with all your mind."

Matthew 22:37
New International Version (NIV)

Dictionary.com defines submit used a verb as to give over or yield to the power or authority or another. Submission, a noun, is an act or instance of submitting or submissive conduct or attitude.

Gage defines submission as giving God back what already belongs to Him.

When women hear or see the words submit and submission, we may think first to a husband and usually within the definition of marriage. While this is true, the first submission required is to God, Christ and Holy Spirit.

Our submission to God is His design. According to Gage, God wants us to be humble enough to submit to Him what belongs to Him:

US. And do so with a <u>willing</u> heart, mind and spirit and body. Our willingness communicates our love and respect to God. Our submission is respectful and honoring of God. The submission is required to continue a relationship with God. God and I cannot both be in charge of me. Only one of us can be in control. God is not going to fight me or compete with me for me. In order for my submission to happen and be AUTHENTIC, I have to submit willingly.

For the purpose of this study, we need to separate yield and submit. Technically they are the same. Biblically, there are some significant differences. Yield is to give over yourself to God. Submit is to give over your will and all of its accessories (pride, ego, work ethic, etc.) to God. The wholeness of your surrender deepens the relationship between you and God.

When we yield to God, we put ourselves in the hand of God. When we submit to God we align ourselves to His will and willingly accept the work He has for us. Yielding is having the correct attitude and spirit. Submitting is doing what God calls you to do with that attitude and spirit.

Both yielding and submitting is required to please God. We spoke of the people who yielded to God in the previous chapter. We noted that because of their yielding, God did great work through them and with them and in response to what they did.

When we consider complete surrender, Jesus is the only person who comes to mind. One may argue that Jesus is not a person. My response is that Jesus was on this Earth and was free from sin for the entirety of His 33 years. The only way to show surrender at its

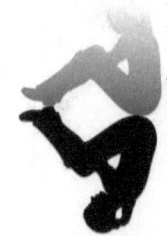

ultimate, definitive practice is to discuss Jesus. Most of us cannot go 33 minutes without a sin. We may go 33 seconds without one, but not 33 hours, not 33 days, not 33 months, and certainly not 33 years. I could count 33 sins and I may cover a four hour time span. That is an average of eight sins each hour.

In describing Jesus as the definition of submissive, Jesus had the power to stop all that happened to Him. He had the power to ask God not to sacrifice Him for us. Yet! He submitted to God and said not My will but Thy will be done. Jesus totally submitted Himself to God. Jesus knew that He would be born, and baptized. He knew he would be preach, teach, perform miracles, walk on water, calm storms, feed the hungry, wash feet, and save lives. He knew He would be betrayed and crucified. And He still did it . . . ALL. ALL of me. For us.

Can we do that for someone else? No, not really! Jesus made an incredible sacrifice. Of which we will never be asked to do.

So when we consider that submission requires sacrifice, we have to ask for help in that regard. We are too weak with pride, guilt and selfishness for submission to be a natural desire. Likewise we will not do it without some comfort and prompting from God.

The benefits of submitting are closer, clearer and consumed faster. A closer relationship with Christ faster. A clearer mind, heart, soul and spirit to hear God with clarity. A consumed-self aligned vessel directed toward God faster. God does fantastic repackaging of His original work after some significant damage of a previous masterpiece.

Our submission is critical to our growth toward God.

Once we submit, we can become completely filled with God's presence.

As you debate the submission concept, I ask you do you trust yourself in the hands of the Creator? Do you trust Him with all of you? Your behavior and attitude says that you do not. The next question is why not? Are you waiting for Him to convince you again that He is God and that you are out of His will when you think you are in charge of yourself?

Our relationship will not be great until we submit.

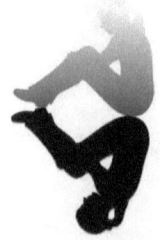

A WOMAN'S JOURNEY FOR A LIFE DEDICATED TO GOD

THE PRAYER FACTOR

Do not be anxious about anything, but in every situation, by prayer and petition, with thanksgiving, present your requests to God.

Philippians 4:6
New International Version (NIV)

Pray without ceasing.

1 Thessalonians 5:17
King James Version (KJV)

[24] Until now you have not asked for anything in my name. Ask and you will receive, and your joy will be complete.

John 16:24
New International Version (NIV)

Every relationship requires communication. The most important relationship we have is between us and God, Jesus and the Holy Spirit. This communication is called prayer. Prayer is the time we spend with God and the Holy Spirit and Jesus are available in the conversation. Prayer is two-way communication. We speak to God. God speaks to us. Prayer is not to be confused with frequently asked questions or question and answer. Also we do not want to confuse this time with a shopping list.

Prayer is a sacred opportunity where we share our hearts with God. God also uses this opportunity where He assumes He has your undivided attention as He should to share His heart and will with you. God will give you much information during prayer. God shares His

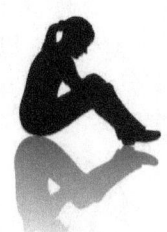

love during prayer. When we pray, we are strengthening our love relationship with Him. Our prayers indicate that the relationship is important to each of us.

In co-facilitating a class with my prayer partner, he posed a question to the class: if God only gave you what you asked for or thanked Him for, what would we have? So we each prayed and at the conclusion, my prayer partner mentioned that none of us had thanked Him for breath that we breathe, healthy bodies, healthy emotional spirits and a stronger relationship with Him. Yet we asked for new "stuff." If we only ask for STUFF in our prayers and do not thank Him for already ample provisions, will we need the STUFF? Will we enjoy the STUFF? What good is a new purse if you don't have an arm on which to carry it?

As we open this dialogue about prayer, I want to remind us that there is not a perfect prayer. Prayer is based on relationship. The more comfortable you are in the relationship, the more you communicate. Also remember that prayer does not guarantee anything! God is sovereign. God's will will be done. His will is not often aligned with the desires of our heart. We want to use that scripture as our override button when God does not give us our way. God's will reaches further than the desires of my heart. As we proceed, consider events in your life that you prayed for something different than what God actually did. Have you discovered why God's will was better than the plans you had? I have several instances, some of which I will share to further illuminate that God's will is **always** best.

Prayer In Scripture

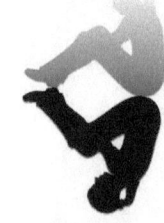

I introduced three scriptures at the opening of this chapter. As we consider those scriptures, I suggest that you find your favorite prayer scriptures. Philippians 4:6 is complete with instructions. Gage's rewrite looks like this: Discard the anxiety about EVERYTHING in our lives. Give EVERYTHING to God in prayer in a respectful and thankful manner. And LEAVE it with Him.

We live in a world where anxiety is rampant. As a Christian and a woman that anxiety can be detrimental to our relationships and our health. As emotional creatures, we are impacted by issues which cause anxiety and we share that through other means. We cannot completely cast our cares on God. This is partially because we "think" we need God to prove to us that He can handle our stuff. We have an event(s) where He did not do what we ask so we subconsciously partitioned our lives from God. We surrender what is out of our reach and we hold on to what we think we can handle ourselves. The truth of the matter is that He can be and He wants to be and should be trusted with it ALL.

When you pray, humbleness and humility is the first order of business. The scripture reads: "with thanksgiving." This means with appreciation. This is a time to remember that you are praying to God. The God who created you and gave you all the titles and stuff which usually support your egotistical and arrogant posture and attitude is the God you are praying to. Bow your head and close your eyes like we did as children. We are His children. He is God! Remember that He is the Source of ALL blessings. If we are able, kneeling would be appropriate as well.

When we pray, God is our Father. There is a respect factor we need to maintain. We are not talking to our friends with whom we work, shop and gossip. While some of us cannot identify with an earthly father, you do have someone you highly respect and your tone, body language, volume, and content exhibit that respect. Likewise, God deserves that same respect.

God designed prayer for us to ASK Him for everything. Ask Him for especially that which we can do for ourselves (or so we think). Thessalonians 5:17 states for us to pray continually. We neglect daily the everything and continually. One of my friends stated to me that she prayed about where and what to eat daily. When she stated that to me, I thought why does she need to pray over something so "small"? The word of God states that we are to seek God in all that we do and need and experience.

How are we to pray continually? Before we speak, pray. Before we do, pray. Before we act, pray. Before we move, pray. To be able to do the continually praying, we have to adjust our mindset about prayer. Prayer is a sacred dialogue between us and God. This conversation can happen anywhere and anytime.

Prayer is essential to our spiritual growth. Prayer is our lifeline to God. Prayer is our air. Our oxygen. Prayer is critical in our decision making. God offers His guidance in our prayers.

In conclusion about the scripture and prayer, God appreciates His word being prayed back to Him as it is relevant to our situation. Reading, understanding and being able to recite His word back to Him communicates your engagement and attentiveness toward God.

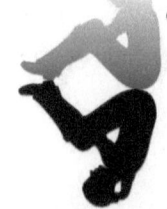

Prayer Timeline

Prayer started with Adam and has evolved several times since then. God talked to Adam and Eve. There was no intermediary. God spoke to Adam and Adam spoke to God. Their actions changed that. When Eve disobeyed, the nature of that dialogue changed.

Prayer was then a dialogue with angel assistance. God chose to communicate in different manners in situations. Often there was an intermediary.

In the New Testament, Jesus became our intermediary. Jesus taught us how to prayer and offered us the use of His name. "If you ask anything in My name, it shall be given you." John 16:24. Jesus introduces the parameters of prayer which we will consider later in this chapter. Then finally, we receive the gift of the Holy Spirit.

The Holy Spirit has quite the job. The Holy Spirit will assist us in prayer. The huge responsibility is not an intermediary but more of a supporter and translator. Likewise, the Holy Spirit intercedes on our behalf when we do not know what to pray.

If prayer was not important to God and our relationship, He would not have given us the use of Jesus' name or the Holy Spirit as an intercessor.

PEOPLE WHO WERE KNOWN TO PRAY

As usual God also gives us examples of who pray, these people serve as examples of what to do in crisis and how to relate to God. In no particular order, Jesus, Paul, David, Jabez, Hannah, and

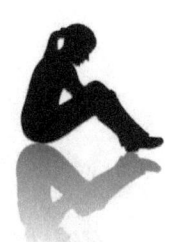

widow of Zeraphath (the woman ready to die). The Bible has prayer warriors. The people take God at His word—unwavering!

The prayer relationship is one they foster and protect. These Christians share how to pray through the storms of life, realize that the storms of life drive us closer to God and strengthen us for the work that God wants us to do.

The lives of those committed servants will share with others for years to come so that their lives will be our roadmap for prayers, answers, activities, actions, and attitudes.

A Special Woman (1 Kings 17:7-24)

The special, unmarried woman had a son, one measure of flour and a portion of oil. This measure of flour and portion of oil was not enough for her and her son to last until Friday. Forgive my pun but in short "until Friday" means that she could not see the provision lasting but another day, maybe two days at the most. Nor did she have a measure a faith for her food lasting to feed them nor did she have any resources to purchase or acquire more. She saw the end of their lives because of this lack of resources. She did not seek other resources. She had reached her own resolve. She would make a final meal and would go to die. What she did not know was that God has her on assignment to feed Elijah with what she had: a handful of flour and a little oil. This is not enough to feed her and her son so certainly it would not feed him as well. But God!

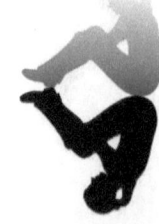

She does not have a measure of faith. When Elijah arrives, she is broken and hurting. God sends Elijah to restore her faith, install her wholeness and prompt her to pray again.

THE PRAYER FACTOR

God chose to use her because He wanted to restore her. Verse 24 reads, "Now I know that you are a man of God and that the word of the Lord from your mouth is the truth."

God planned for her restoration. The text does not state that she prayed at any point. The text reveals her disbelief and obedience with her disbelief in place. When God filled her jars with flour and oil, the filling was not enough to restore her faith or cause her to pray or believe. If it were one of us, we would have stopped short of the blessings God planned for us by doubting, and even quitting. A few of us would not even let Elijah in our homes. We would not allow him nor would we have trusted enough to open our homes or hearts to be blessed the way God planned through Elijah.

God uses events and people to drives us back to Him. He created us to worship Him; a part of that worship is prayer.

Hannah—The Ideal Mother (1 Samuel 1:2-11)

Hannah had a life other woman did not envy until the Lord showed up and delivered His promises to Hannah. Hannah could not have children for the first several years of her marriage. Her husband had another wife who had children. The other woman provoked her and rubbed it in that she does not have children. During this time, children and child birth validated a woman as a woman in the public eye. So Hannah is feeling less than a woman and she appeals to God. Verse 7 reads that Hannah wept and would not eat. Her husband did not understand her emptiness yet attempted to console her saying that "don't I mean more to you than ten sons?" in verse 8.

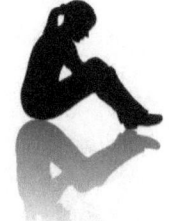

YIELDED AND SUBMITTED

Hannah diligently seeks God. She was suffering from a bitter soul. Hannah prayed fervently to God, pleading with God to open her womb and validate her womanhood. Verse 11 is the deal of lifetime. Hannah PROMISES God that if He gives her a son, she will give him back to God immediately for all of the days of her life.

Eli observed her prayer and he blessed her and agreed with her, asking God to grant her request. Hannah was granted the son she requested. Hannah upheld her part of the PROMISE. Hannah brought her son to Eli and reminded him of whom she was. She left her gift: her son; just as she said she would.

Hannah is powerful example of prayer. She was not afraid to seek God for her desires. She was honest with God and direct toward Him. Hannah has an authentic worship toward God. She trusted God with her needs and desires. She was grateful for her husband's favor (verse 5) but a son would make her complete.

Hannah's prayers were incessant and consistent. Hannah did not waiver in her prayer to God. She considered her persistence a valuable trait before God. She prayed whether she was understood or not. She prayed diligently. She was intent on proving to God she was worthy of her request.

Hannah was passionate about her request to God. She prayed with expression and emotion. She was not dry or pretentious. She expressed herself to God. She did not hide her feelings from God.

Hannah was transparent about her needs and prayers. She shared openly with her husband and Eli her requests from God. Hannah openly asked God and expected Him to fulfill her request. Hannah

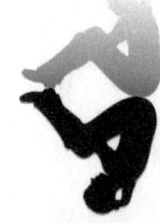

states to Eli: "I have been praying here out of my great anguish and grief." Verse 16b.

Hannah makes the deal of a lifetime with God. Many of us make deals with God and never keep them. God believes Hannah will keep her word. God blessed her to conceive. Hannah's faith never wanes during this time. She is faithful to God.

When Hannah presents this powerful proposal, God is the one who takes the risk. When God decides to grants her request, she is faithful. She rejoices for God's gift. Hannah names her son Samuel, saying, "Because I asked God for him." (verse 20).

Hannah honors God through keeping her promise. She prepares Samuel for his life before God. She delivers him to Eli with a sacrifice to God. God is honored by her dedication and commitment. God receives Samuel and the sacrifice she brought.

Hannah shares her testimony in an humble and authentic manner which I believe even moves Eli. She passionately reminds Eli who she is and shares God's favor with Eli (verses 26-28).

Hannah does not weep over her gift and sacrifice. She brings Samuel joyfully to Eli to serve and worship for the rest of his life.

God honors her actions and humility by blessing her with seven more children who she raised at home. Hannah spends the first eleven verses of chapter two praying more to God. She shares her rejoice and delight in delivery above her enemies. She praises and worships God for His holiness. She cautions us not to be arrogant and prideful, which will not get past God. She explains the power, strength and ability of God. She recalls the emotional state of her enemy.

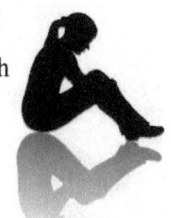

Hannah already had her husband's favor and now it was probably greater because her countenance had changed because of the overwhelming favor of God. Her husband was also honored by her attitude about the entire situation. Hannah never negatively addressed his other wife when she was unkind to Hannah. Hannah warns against the perception of strength to prevail in matters rather than the will of God.

Hannah unequivocally shares the far-reaching authority of God.

Hannah teaches us so much about prayer. Hannah challenges us to remain focused on God to stay focused on what God says and is doing and what He wants. Hannah is faithful and never questions God. Hannah does not give up on God not matter how long it takes.

Hannah teaches us that we may pray the same prayer until God answers. Please do not get confused with His answer being always equal to the desire of your heart. He may not give you what you want, but what you receive will be best for you.

Hannah was willing to sacrifice her gift completely, and without regret to God. She made a deal with God and kept her part of the bargain.

Hannah's humility brought her blessings. She did not forget the Lord wanted her to be someone He could trust inside of the entire circumstance. We may find ourselves wanting to retaliate. Avoid that desire because retaliation will offend God. We need to remember God wants to trust us. Our negative behavior will erode that possibility. God creates in us the ability to worship and praise Him. This worship and

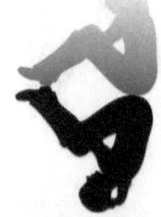

praise needs to be consistent through that season. God wants us to be transparent about what God is doing and has done in our lives. Most of the time we are not authentic, nor completely honest and not nearly transparent enough to offer God any real part of ourselves.

God blesses those who will speak on God's behalf for what He has done in our lives. Most Christians do not want to share our struggles so it makes it hard to share God's work. Without this transparency, God may be reluctant to offer you the desires of your heart. Without sharing the circumstances, when the blessing comes, it seems like a bonus when it is really the solution where God will probably not get the glory He planned and deserves. When we don't tell the whole story our testimony is weakened. God's glory is downplayed.

We need to abandon the concern that we need to manage who we can trust with our testimonies. What happens to us and how God chooses to resolve our issues are the total ownership and responsibility of God. God chooses who needs that testimony and we are not at liberty to change that plan. Improperly sharing, whether to the wrong person or in an incomplete manner, serves to delay God's purpose. That testimony is designed to exhibit God to others who are in need of that experience. When we do not share correctly, we modify their vision and understanding of God and possibly cause confusion in them for what God already shared and showed them.

Hannah demonstrates the benefit of transparency. As a result of her transparency, Eli was able to agree with her prayer and offer her a blessing. Eli witnessed her sincerity and he offered his confidence for God's favor within her life.

Hannah loves God. Hannah does not lie nor does she hide from God. Prayer is the way to God. God tested her heart and its commitment to God. Hannah teaches so much but here we focused on prayer. I am certain there were days where she may have wanted to see him or maybe even missed him but I doubt she ever regretted what she did. I would believe that God's peace filled that space bountifully.

Because of her prayers, faith and sincerity, she birthed one of the greatest servants God ever had. Is your mediocre or absent or arrogant prayer life blocking and delaying blessings for this or future generations?

David (1 Samuel, 2 Samuel, Psalm)

David, a man after God's own heart, molded in God's very image and the king who other's model, admire, and study closely. David's life starts our modestly enough and visits plenty of peaks. For our study of prayer we will go directly to the prayer after Nathan's visit to him where Nathan reveals that God is unhappy with him: 2 Samuel 12:15-23.

David had sinned. Because of that sin, a son was born. That son was struck ill because of that sin. In his repentance for that sin, David admitted his sin, prayed and fervently fasted for seven days, until the child died. David did what he felt the Lord wanted. David knew the son would die before he prayed and fasted. David hoped that his repented behavior would change the heart of God. The child still died.

We do not always get the desires of our hearts. Sometimes God says no, like in this case. God's no does not indicate He does not

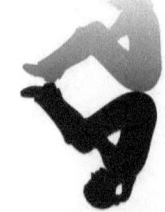

love us. Instead He communicates that we are loved yet we are sinners and there are consequences to those sins.

David's sins did not stop God from blessing him. David went to Bathsheba to comfort her and they conceived Solomon. David was blessed to birth the next king. David had to be punished for he had sinned out of greed. David could have asked for Bathsheba or chosen someone else. David misused his power as king which was given by God. God was absolute when He sent Nathan to David share His anger.

David teaches us to pray mightily ESPECIALLY when our situation looks bleak. Our fervent prayer MAY change His heart. Even if it does not, it is what His word says to do.

David introduced us to fasting within the context of our study. When we fast, we are giving up something sacrificially in order to offer ourselves more focused and pure to God. Fasting on a regular basis and for matters which you are hoping for God's special attention is beneficial. Fasting is a purifying experience. Fasting eliminates distractions—especially those who keep us from God. Prayer warriors fast regularly and present their requests and petitions to God.

When fasting, fasting should not be shared unless with a prayer partner or for medical purposes. I recall being in a difficult work situation. I fasted weekly on Thursday and I prayed mightily. God was faithful and gracious. God gave me a solution but not quite the one I had planned.

David did not receive the answer for which he hoped, however, when that ended differently, David did not frown or pout or sulk. He was told the baby died, he comforted Bathsheba, conceived

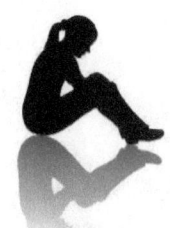

Solomon and went to war. He returned to his duties as king. Part of pleasing God is accepting His answers as they are. His answers are non-negotiable.

David also reminds us to pray continually. I am just guessing that David did not pray before the decision he made which was the source of this trouble anyway. When he did not start out praying, he did not seek God about his desires. The risk is that we have excluded God from huge life-changing events. David did not ask God if Bathsheba was right for him or many other things, most importantly for forgiveness of his sins. He never asked God to forgive him. Prayer allows time for God to reveal to us the aspects and details we overlook but still require His attention and our dialogue. David now was forgiven for that sin and situation.

David spends extensive time with God through prayer in the book of Psalm. David prays to God regularly. David completely shares his heart and is profoundly transparent. David compels us to be transparent and trusting of God completely.

Saul (Acts 9)

Saul was transformed into Paul, one of the greatest preachers, theologians, apostles who ever lived. Paul prayed. Paul prayed over everyone and everywhere. Paul's prayers are some of the most profound prayers in the Bible.

Paul's prayers host many lessons, of which we will discuss two prayers, which are my favorite because of their power. Paul is the active voice and author of Romans, 1 & 2 Corinthians, Galatians, Ephesians, Philippians, Colossians, 1 & 2 Thessalonians, 1 & 2

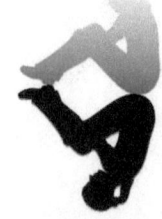

Timothy, Titus, and Philemon—a total of 13 books of the new testament, almost half of the new testament. Paul was originally Saul in Acts. Saul's transformation into Christianity was profound and definite. When Saul became a Christian, he was also immediately a preacher. Saul understood and answered the call of God immediately.

As Christians, most of us debate with God about what He means or what exactly He says and how that affects us and our lives. Saul became Paul in spite of the criticisms because of his past when he stood BOLDLY against Jesus.

The letters of Paul always opens praising, worshipping and praying to God. Paul is always thankful to God for the opportunity to serve Jesus.

My favorite two prayers are 2 Corinthians 12:7-10 and Ephesians 3:14-21. Paul shares his heart with all those in his reach. Paul is not discriminatory in sharing his message and his heart is full of compassion.

2 Corinthians 12:7-10, Paul was given a thorn in his side. Paul recognizes that the thorn is designed to keep him humble and so that he does not boast about what the Lord has done as though it was his own doing.

[7] To keep me from becoming conceited because of these surpassingly great revelations, there was given me a thorn in my flesh, a messenger of Satan, to torment me. [8] Three times I pleaded with the Lord to take it away from me. [9] But he said to me, "My grace is sufficient for you, for my power is made perfect in weakness." Therefore I will boast all the more gladly about my weaknesses, so that

YIELDED AND SUBMITTED

Christ's power may rest on me. [10] That is why, for Christ's sake, I delight in weaknesses, in insults, in hardships, in persecutions, in difficulties. For when I am weak, then I am strong.

Paul stood and asked God for comfort and consideration for the thorn which was in his side. God said I will not remove it but I will offer you My grace as you carry it. Keep in mind that God does not owe us anything, especially not an answer to prayer. God reminded Paul that My power is so much more evident when you are weak.

Paul's plea was well presented to God. Paul was authentic. Paul understands the Source of His relief. Paul has submitted himself totally to God. Paul teaches the value of authentic prayer rather than the perfunctory prayers similar to the laws he advises against.

My second favorite is Ephesians 3:14-21.

[14] For this reason I kneel before the Father, [15] from whom His whole family[a] in heaven and on earth derives its name. [16] I pray that out of His glorious riches He may strengthen you with power through His Spirit in your inner being, [17] so that Christ may dwell in your hearts through faith. And I pray that you, being rooted and established in love, [18] may have power, together with all the saints, to grasp how wide and long and high and deep is the love of Christ, [19] and to know this love that surpasses knowledge —that you may be filled to the measure of all the fullness of God. [20] Now to Him who is able to do immeasurably more than all we ask or imagine, according to His power that is at work within us, [21] to Him be glory in the church and in Christ Jesus throughout all generations, forever and ever! Amen.

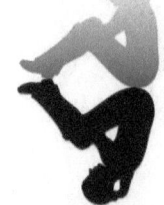

Paul prays for the church of Ephesus and by extension you and I. This intercessory prayer moved and changed my heart. These verses have been the foundation for many sermons. Paul prays from the heart. He does not use fancy transitions or convoluted jargon to speak to God or share what God said with us. Paul shares with us sound doctrine and instructions from God which we should follow and understand the nature of His messages.

Because of the weight of this prayer, these are some of my favorite scriptures. In his prayer, he shares with us some quite affirming statements. When he prays for my strength of my inner being with the power of the Holy Spirit, I shudder. When he reminds me that Christ dwells in my heart through faith, I am so humbled. Paul stirs my soul when he prays that I am rooted in established in love—God's unconditional love—and nothing can change that love regardless of how I mess up or what others say or do. He prays for me to have power to understand the measure of God's love. When he shares the infinite measure of God's love and that ALL of it is mine: I weep. Uncontrollably. When Paul prays for me to be full of the measure which surpasses my mini-understanding, which COMPLETELY replaces the emptiness I could feel at any time because of my temporary situation.

Finally, Paul closes the prayer reminding me by offering glory to God that God can do more than what I can think of, dream about, consider, ponder, wonder about question and imagine and so much more! This is all because His power is at work within me. Paul offers me wisdom when he prays, particularly in the last statement when he reminds me that I have to surrender to God's power so that He can work within me.

I am moved when Paul intercedes for me as well as when others intercede for me. It is humbling and profound.

Paul is a prayer warrior. He shares the gift with us. Paul teaches us that the power of prayer exists within all of us. Paul confirms the word of God with his actions. He urges us to be diligent about our prayers of God in Jesus' name paired with the power of the Holy Spirit.

Paul causes us to ask the following questions:

- Do we pray fervently?
- Do we pray authentically?
- Do we pray with a clean heart?
- Do we pray for others?
- Do we openly share with others the needs we have so that we can also intercede on each other's behalf?
- Do we pray consistently?
- How do we lead others to God?

As we address these questions, we should grow closer to Christ through prayer. Paul leads us to that closer growth.

Jesus Christ the King

Jesus Christ our King teaches us how to pray. He serves as our ultimate example for prayer. First, He teaches us to pray is Matthew 6:5-15. Secondly, He models prayer for us. Thirdly, He experiences prayer and submission to God's will. Finally, Jesus left us a gift to facilitate our prayers as an extension of Him and an intercessor.

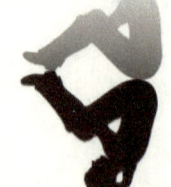

Jesus teaches us to pray through His words in Matthew 6:5-15.

⁵ "And when you pray, do not be like the hypocrites, for they love to pray standing in the synagogues and on the street corners to be seen by men. I tell you the truth, they have received their reward in full. ⁶ But when you pray, go into your room, close the door and pray to your Father, who is unseen. Then your Father, who sees what is done in secret, will reward you. ⁷ And when you pray, do not keep on babbling like pagans, for they think they will be heard because of their many words. ⁸ Do not be like them, for your Father knows what you need before you ask him. ⁹ "This, then, is how you should pray: "'Our Father in heaven, hallowed be your name, ¹⁰ your kingdom come, your will be done on earth as it is in heaven.

¹¹ Give us today our daily bread.

¹² Forgive us our debts, as we also have forgiven our debtors.

¹³ And lead us not into temptation, but deliver us from the evil one.[a],

¹⁴ For if you forgive men when they sin against you, your heavenly Father will also forgive you. ¹⁵ But if you do not forgive men their sins, your Father will not forgive your sins.

Prayer guidelines:

1. Do not pray to be seen.
2. Pray to God in a room, behind a closed door.
3. In secret, God will reward you.
4. Do not go on and on. The multiple, repetitive words do not impress God.
5. Do not lie when you pray. Do not omit anything from God. He already knows what we need.
6. Pray with sincerity.
7. Pray with humility and meekness.

8. Thank God for the essentials of daily bread.
9. Acknowledge God's holiness.
10. Acknowledge that God's will be done. Everywhere.
11. Request to be forgiven for our sins.
12. Request to be able to avoid temptation.

These twelve guidelines are not comprehensive, yet rather a start for what a prayer to God really includes and what our prayers weigh.

Jesus has a significant prayer life obviously. There are some specific events we will cover, three of which is about His prayer life: The Last Supper, The Garden of Gethsemane and On the Cross.

Before we consider these prayers, I wish we would consider the instances where there was no obvious praying but prayer had to exist. Jesus prayed mightily during the Forty day fast. Those prayers had to be mighty because Jesus would not make it without prayer.

Jesus healed many for the purpose of sharing who He is for them. These miracles required prayer. Everyone has an ailment and an illness and a need. He had to choose exactly the persons who would share Him with others. Some of us are not healed, delivered and are not receiving His immediate attention in that manner because we cannot be trusted to share or we will take the glory away from God.

Jesus had to pray more than is obvious in the Bible. He is the example of an honest and transparent relationship with God. For this to happen, prayer is required. There are examples of non-obvious yet quite evident praying.

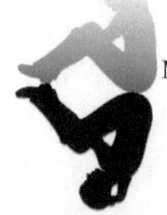

Jesus prays over The Lord's Supper. Verse 26, chapter 26 of Matthew reads [He] gave thanks. Verse 27, chapter 26 of Matthew,

Jesus again gave thanks. After Jesus gave thanks, Jesus explains what they will consume and what the bread and the drink means. This moment of thanksgiving is one of the most important prayers ever given. This prayer is inclusive of a commitment to the covenant of Christ.

The powerful works which Jesus speaks initiated an experience most Christians do each month that is referred to as Communion and the Lord's Supper. This intimate encounter is still regarded as high now as it was then, maybe more so now.

As we recall this prayer, which is not detailed but only referred to as giving thanks, we are reminded to be thankful to God. A prayer of thanks is the measure of what God does for us and how we appreciate Him. One of my favorite songs says that God gets happy when we just say thank you. I do not know true that is but I do know that there is a human need we have to be appreciated so I am sure that God would like the experience as well. As Jesus teaches us to say thank You to God in prayer, we are reminded that we are not self-made, nor self-sustaining. We are not independent of God. Our thankfulness demonstrates that we understand that. God deserves our authentic gratitude.

Jesus prays at the Garden of Gethsemane. Jesus is preparing for His crucifixion. He has a heavy heart because He has just shared the Last Supper and predicts Peter's denial of Him and most importantly, Judas' betrayal. He goes to God because He is sorrowful and is seeking God's comfort. Jesus asks God to take this 'cup' away from Him. Jesus lay prostrate before God which exhibits His ultimate commitment to God and to God's will.

He prays that some other provision would be made but does not negotiate with God and submits to His ultimate will. Jesus does understand the weight of His duty and the fulfillment of the scripture. This did not make it easier for Jesus to accept. Jesus PRAYED. God did not change the PLAN. God may have appeared to say no to Jesus but in the fulfillment of the scripture said yes to so much more. Jesus humbly submits His requests to God.

God makes the final decision.

As Jesus prays, He asks the disciples to "keep watch." Keep watch means to stay awake and attentive while Jesus prays. The disciples should have been praying as well. They should have at the minimum been reflecting on the events which have previously transpired. Jesus shared with them the coming events and they are not concerned or consumed with the gravity of the events.

As co-laborers with Jesus Christ, we likewise should "keep watch" over the affairs which concern Jesus and the work we were left and designed to complete. As disciples, we are designed to reach others to bring others to Christ and share more of Christ's teachings with others. We are to pray, fast, teach, preach, evangelize, and use our spiritual gifts in a manner where Jesus is glorified and manifested. Effective use of our gifts translates into the wisdom to behave wisely in God's eyes, guide others to Christ so that others will experience the only unconditional love they will ever experience, and understanding the God who created us in such a profound manner that we stand for God and NEVER doubt.

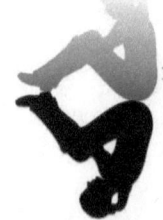

When we "keep watch," we also intercede for others. Less mature and new Christians and non-Christians look to you for answers, information, wisdom, and faithful behavior. When we do not do these things, we cause doubt in their minds. We often ask ourselves why won't 'they' come to Christ, not knowing the answer is "because of us and our lack of faith and questionable behavior."

Our prayer life is important to remain connected to Christ. Jesus teaches us this by example not by talking about it. This particular request is so serious; more serious than other requests ever made. Jesus asks to be excused from saving us from our sins! Aren't you happy God said no? I know that I am. This is what we need to remember when God says no. His "no" means so much more than we can understand initially. His "no" to Jesus saved my sorry, sinful soul. There are times when He has told you 'no' and He saved you from yourself.

Jesus shows us the power of prayer in John 17. Jesus prays for us to God in a direct manner that God protects us from the evil one. Jesus' tone is conversational and respectful. Jesus prays God's words back to Him. Jesus shares His heart with God about us. Jesus prays with a spectacular compassion because of His love for us. Jesus is praying to our Creator sharing how He wants no harm to come to us but to prosper us and comfort us. There are those of us who fall under this very prayer and protection who do not understand how Jesus' love could still exist even though we have wronged Him because of sin and disobedience.

Jesus approaches God on our behalf with the unconditional love that only God provides. As we consider the details of His prayer, we have to understand what it means when He said we were His

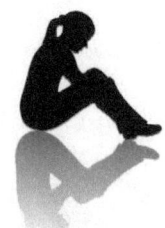

friends, when He came to offer us eternal life because of salvation, and when He defined love for us.

When Jesus prays, consider the following: what Jesus said to God, what Jesus did and what we do in response.

If only we could pray like Jesus, but since we cannot, we should pray daily, diligently and reverently.

The Prayer of Jabez (1 Chronicles 4:9-10)

⁹ Jabez was more honorable than his brothers. His mother had named him Jabez,[a] saying, "I gave birth to him in pain." ¹⁰ Jabez cried out to the God of Israel, "Oh, that you would bless me and enlarge my territory! Let your hand be with me, and keep me from harm so that I will be free from pain." And God granted his request.

Who is Jabez? Who is his mother? What was Jabez's territory? Why does he want that territory enlarged? Why does he seek God? Why does God grant his request? Who does the enlargement benefit? What was the far reaching effect of the prayer and the answer God gives? I pose these questions because we need to understand the power of prayer and the heart of God, when we pray. Not much is known about Jabez however the most powerful point is that he prayed and God answered. He granted Jabez his request.

The first thing we know about Jabez is that he was honorable, more so than his brothers. The honorability of Jabez probably impressed God. In our daily lives our siblings have a powerful influence over us. The fact that Jabez avoided their foolish activities and escaped their persuasion meant something to God. He may have proven to God that he was trustworthy of God's blessings.

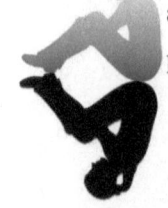

THE PRAYER FACTOR

Jabez made three requests, one of which is well known but the second two, we will investigate first. Jabez asked for God's protection from harm and pain. Likewise, Jabez asked for God's hand be with him. This could mean His hand to protect, to guide, or/and to provide. He grants them all! The significance of the requests of protection from harm and pain were so bold and perhaps the request for guidance was so unique that God decided on the worth of the request being granted and the requestor.

As God considers our requests, are we worthy of that request being granted? No. I do not need to know what the request is or why you want it or what it will do for you. We simply do not DESERVE anything we request.

We are granted requests because God is gracious. He considers our requests compared to His will and decides whether that request is feasible to grant or better to deny. His granting or denial is subject to His revocation. The denial may be temporary so that God will grant on a delayed time frame. The granting of this provision can be later denied.

God granted Jabez's request because God and God alone makes this decision and it is not up for debate.

The last request was to enlarge his territory. God does not give more to those who are not managing well that which they are already responsible. If you are not managing what God already given you well, it is unlikely that He will give you more. It is likely that Jabez had managed his smaller territory well—so well that God gave him more.

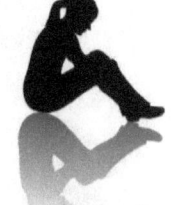

God expects us to pray and understand He answers and His decision is what is best for each of us at the time. God considers our character and our responsiveness to Him and His will important when making decisions.

Who Me? Pray? Out Loud? Wow!

Yes, You! Yes, pray out loud. No wow necessary. When I was invited to pray in front of a group for the first time, I wondered what I would pray about. The Holy Spirit offered two declarations: (1) You are not praying to them. You are praying to HIM! And, (2) I am with you when you do not know what to pray for.

I love to pray for others. I am never anxious to pray for others but I know that I have the gift to intercede for others. Because of what I am charged with, I make myself available as often as I can. The prayer critique though is that I speak so softly sometimes that others cannot hear my prayer. I am really not talking to them. While that may be true, I need the others in the circle to agree with me. As a collective, we serve God and for that reason I try to pray so that others may agree with me before God for the needs, and pleas of His people.

If this is a real fear for you, then start out loud in your quiet time when you are alone. Next, pray over the meals. Then have family prayer. Family prayer is the hardest because it involves transparency. As the adult of the home, you have to be transparent first. This means being genuine and authentic in front of your children and spouse. It is my prayer that you will be the transforming component in your family. I pray that you share your deepest thoughts, your heaviest concerns and your family secrets when you pray.

THE PRAYER FACTOR

Tell your children that you are concerned about their grades, about the influence their friends may have over them, about drug use, and about sex. When you are honest with them, they can then be honest with you. Share with them what your school experience was like so that they understand your expectations. When you share your experiences, good, bad and indifferent, they can better understand what is needed to be successful and keep you happy. As an educator, what I have learned is that they do not understand you as a parent or person. They have said that as parents you do not share enough with them. Also, having watched many parent-child interactions, I have concluded that you are secretly hoping for their success but you are not willing to share how to achieve that desired success.

This all started about family prayer. This is a key for family success. Family prayer is about the family unit. With so many units taking on different shapes and meanings. Whatever defines your family structure, the key is to pray for it with your family. There is power in transparency. Several students taught me that.

I have learned so much about my family through other means than my family's transparency. It was embarrassing and horrible. You can avoid that problem if you just share it yourself. Also be reminded that any public information about you and your family can be found on the internet. How would you like to be confronted about your family "secrets" on the internet?

Anyway, family prayer is key. Share the responsibilities of prayer. Have a place for prayer requests and praise reports. A board or basket could be used. This is an opportunity to share without a verbal

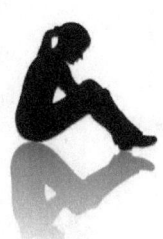

sharing. This is key for hard-to-say requests. Closeness should result from the prayers of your family.

Finally, when the children pray at home, they will pray confidently out loud in public later in life.

Pray now so that they can pray later.

What Does God Expect from My Prayers?

God has requested our honest, consistent and genuine prayers. God expects us to have daily and regularly meaningful dialogue with Him about our lives which most of the time is defined as sheer foolishness. Daily and regularly are different. Daily is everyday. Regularly is throughout the day. God expects our honesty. God knows your thoughts before you pray so being dishonest by commission or omission is still lying to yourself and to God. Lying to yourself and trying to lie to God is inefficient for overcoming your issues or getting your needs met. Why not tell Him what He already knows anyway? I am aware of the pain involved in telling God how you feel and what you need. I am aware of the pain of confessing your pain to God. I am aware of the pain of hearing our pains, issues, and fears out loud. I am aware of how hard it is to tell God your sins out loud because you have to remember what you did in order to confess it and you have to confess that you really did THAT!

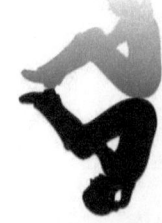

Prayer with God should develop into a respectful dialogue with your best friend. Your dialogue should be authentic and respectful; reverent and genuine; talkative and silent. Prayer is a dialogue not a monologue. Prayer is a two-way communication. We share with God. God shares with us. God wants to hear our cares, our tears, our smiles, our laughter, and our pain. He is waiting on our thanksgiving, adoration, confession and supplication. After all that, God then shares with us His will, His ways and His answers. God shares with me His heart. God tells me how He's pleased and displeased with me. God tells me the place He wants me to stand and walk; run and jump. God plans for me and keeps me safe. God tells me how He cares for me and that He has His hands on me. There are times when God is silent. There are times when we will be silent together while in prayer.

God expects us to listen to Him AND do what He says. God expects us to depend fully and completely on HIM. And ONLY Him. God offers us healing for our ailments. God offers us rest from our burdens. God expects our love. God expects us to understand that He is not our cosmic bell-hop. God's will prevails regardless of what we want. God is going to do His will in our lives and what we want needs to fit within God's plans.

God needs us to realize that His will is that most important aspect of the relationship, meaning we cannot get mad when we do not get what we ask, when we want it, how we want it or when God says no or wait. God has a timing by which He determines if we are ready for what we ask.

God expects us to accept His answers. Our understanding of His work is not required. He knows which of us are going to question His decisions, however from one questioner to another, PROCEED WITH CAUTION. When I have asked God, 'why me?' even in my humble prayer voice, God's response has been, 'Why not you, Onedia?' God is going to strengthen us for His plans so that we may execute His will accordingly. So that we may be strong and equipped

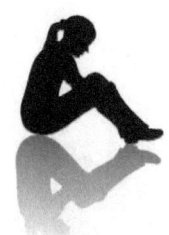

for what He needs for us to do, we need to be strong. God's will, plan, and desires for us are not for the weak or faint at heart. God's plan, will and work requires a strong person—a strength only He can provide.

Lastly, God expects us to pray for others as well. God expects us not to be selfish. We need to support others on this Christian journey. Prayer is the first step for that help for others who need our wisdom for their journey.

Prayer is nourishment for our inner most parts.

What Should I Expect From God

I can expect

- Answers
- Comfort
- Peace
- Love
- Forgiveness
- Patience
- Impatience
- Confirmation
- Discipline
- Strength
- The fruit of the spirit
- Guidance
- Directions
- Memory recall
- Discernment
- Knowledge

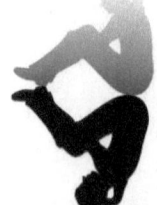

- Grace
- Mercy

Prayer Rules and Etiquette

Prayer is not new by any means. Prayer has changed over many centuries. So the "rules" we have and the "etiquette" are not as current as we may want to understand.

At the very basis of prayer: humility and reverence. We are addressing God, not our best friend or parent or boss. Both of these are based on releasing the attitude and the understanding who God is. This also speaks to posture, a bowed head, closed eyes and an humbled heart.

The "old days" reported on your knees but this is universal. Paul shares in Ephesians 3:14 "I kneel before you." While Paul is not seen as the ultimate on prayer in the New Testament, he is in my top three if I were labeling prayer warriors, mentors and instructors. Jesus is first. John the Baptist is second.

An humble heart is defined as understanding that we are not worthy of anything God gifts us with. NOTHING. If God does not do anything else for me, I would have to be okay with that because I already have more than I deserve. An humble heart also means that we accept what He says, gives and disciplines us with. An humble heart means that we thank God for what He is doing in our lives. An humble heart means that we realize that God uses ALL of our circumstances to bring His glory. An humble heart defines our relationship with God. An humble heart means that God is truly Lord of your life. An humble heart lacks arrogance, confidence and haughtiness. An humble heart houses love, compassion, long-suffering, patience, kindness, meekness, forgiveness, peace, faith, and goodness. An humble heart seeks God's will and aligns our lives to His will. An humble heart puts our selfishness aside. An humble heart gratefully receives what God has for us which is so much better and so much fuller than what we could think up on our own.

After we demonstrate reverence, humbleness, the fruit of the spirit and humility, then we need to understand God's love toward us—the unconditional love He created. We then need to demonstrate a willingness to submit to God's will. Once we demonstrate that, we can seek Him authentically and genuinely.

When we abandon our selfishness, we can actually receive God's intended blessings. Some of us pray to God as if we are doing God a favor. Some of us make deals with God. We start our prayers with "God, if You do _____, then I'll do _____ _____." That is not a prayer and God is not that type of negotiator. Some of us take God for granted. Some pray when we need something. Some of us expect God to answer us immediately rather than in His pre-planned time for WHATEVER His reasons are.

God is sovereign. God is all-knowing. OMNIPOTENT. OMNISCIENT. OMNIPRESENT.

Jesus introduces us to the "rules" which state to not babble on and on like those who have wavering faith. Jesus also demonstrates how to pray with the understanding that we do not have the last word.

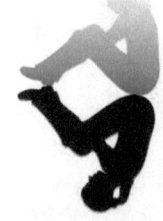

Jesus fasted for the crucifixion to be removed from His responsibility yet submitted to God's will although He knew the pain

He would endure to fulfill God's will. Just as a side note, I have often thought if I only know what would happen next or several steps ahead then this life would be better. The truth is that if I actually knew, I would be trying to change that as well.

Jesus also offers us the opportunity to be granted the desires of our heart within the will of God based on if two or more are gathered in Jesus' name, if we pray if Jesus' name, and if we delight ourselves in Him.

Jesus prays several times, one of which we have labeled as The Lord's Prayer. Luke 6:9-13, Jesus covers the "components" of prayer. The most important aspect of prayer is truth. Jesus could have omitted the part of "if this cup could be removed" but He shared it anyway because He was talking to God.

Jesus truly valued prayer and showed us how to do the same.

The Ultimate Gift in Prayer: The Holy Spirit

God is the best planner for our lives! He already anticipated the best argument we could create: I don't know what to prayer for. Jesus gifted us with the Holy Spirit. John 14 shares with us the promise of the Holy Spirit.

[15] "If you love me, you will obey what I command. [16] And I will ask the Father, and He will give you another Counselor to be with you forever— [17] the Spirit of truth. The world cannot accept Him, because it neither sees Him nor knows Him. But you know Him, for He lives with you and will be in you.

Romans 8:25-27 reads [25] But if we hope for what we do not yet have, we wait for it patiently. [26] In the same way, the Spirit helps us in our weakness. We do not know what we ought to pray for, but the Spirit himself intercedes for us with groans that words cannot express. [27] And he who searches our hearts knows the mind of the Spirit, because the Spirit intercedes for the saints in accordance with God's will.

The Holy Spirit is designed to intercede on our behalf. God puts us in a place to also intercede for others. Jesus gave Him as a gift because Jesus was leaving us.

The Power of a Prayer Partner

[19] "Again, I tell you that if two of you on earth agree about anything you ask for, it will be done for you by my Father in heaven. [20] For where two or three come together in my name, there am I with them." Matthew 18:19-20.

There's comfort and accountability built into that relationship where prayer is that primary focus. Prayer partners pray together in the presence of God. They remind each other what they have prayed for and keep watch over one another. This person is someone who can be trusted with your expressions, confessions and adoration. This person may receive guidance from God, Jesus and the Holy Spirit for you and your situation. You may as well for your partner.

With prayer partners, trust is paramount. What happens during prayer stays in prayer. Transparency is also critical. I have prayed with people and realized that they were not being transparent so I stopped praying with them. Transparency is based on relationship and you are creating a relationship in front of God. That transparency is needed for

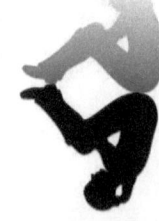

the growth toward God. Your testimony is beneficial and necessary for the growth of others. Keep in mind that you could be withholding valuable information from your prayer partner that they need to handle their situation. When we are not transparent, we can block someone's blessings. This is not what God intends for you or your partner.

You are both accountable EQUALLY.

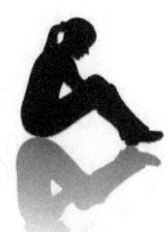

YIELDED AND SUBMITTED

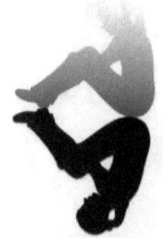

A WOMAN'S JOURNEY FOR A LIFE DEDICATED TO GOD

THE FAITH FACTOR

And without faith it is impossible to please God, because anyone who comes to Him must believe that He exists and that He rewards those who earnestly seek Him.

Hebrews 11:6
New International Version (NIV)

November, 2008, Nehemiah, my son had a perpetual nose bleed. His nose was bleeding daily for several days. On Wednesday before Thanksgiving, I went to the emergency room. They ran test after test. At some point during the night, they placed us in a room. I really did not know what was wrong with my baby. Well, I finally left the room for a few minutes and went to the lounge. Upon looking around the walls and then specifically in the break room, I realized we were on the oncology floor for children! I panicked.

I was devastated! I would have never imagined in forever that I would have been in the cancer center at Texas Children's Hospital in Houston, TX, with my three year old son. I immediately returned to pray with my son. I prayed over him. I cried over him. I returned him to God. I stood on my faith that God had a plan. The final test before we were released was the bone marrow biopsy. They were going to take a bone marrow sample to test for leukemia. My son was being tested for leukemia! After all of that, they released us home. Two days later, I got the call that he did not have leukemia. I cried. I praised the Lord. I wailed before the Lord.

I realized that my faith had been tested. "What will she do in this storm? Under these conditions? In this situation? Will she share her experience with others expressing how God did miraculous measures in her life? How will she learn from this experience? How will this increase her relationship with God?"

Where is your faith? How much does it take to shake your faith? A little storm or a hurricane? In this life, stuff will happen. STUFF is an acronym for situations that unravel your faith and future. When we give in to those situations, we demonstrate a lack of faith. When we demonstrate a lack of faith, we tell God that He is not able to care for us like He promised and has repeatedly demonstrated that He is capable. We tell God that our problems are bigger than His ability and beyond His plan. When we do not exercise faith, we tell God that we do not really believe that faith is important or God's promises are real.

Faith is an intrical part of our Christianity. As a Christian, others measure our Christianity by our faith. When we sound and respond exactly like a non-believer, then what does Christianity really mean? Faith is the definition of Christianity. This is the explanation of Christianity.

Why is faith required of Christians? Christianity communicates to God that we believe He exists and that He is on your side, with plans for you to prosper, regardless of your situation. You may be thinking I am faithful. You may very well be faithful. The challenge we have is CONSISTENT faith. Faith in all situations! The truth is that we do not have consistent faith. During the brief season of Nehemiah's illness, I doubted God. I also questioned God. My questions were not 'What do You want me to learn' and 'What am I to learn.' My questions were more like 'Why me, God? Why my baby?' This line of questioning expresses the lack of faith that I had at that moment. Does this last long? Not really but any lack of faith is really unacceptable. You may ask why is that? Our exercise of faith is also a demonstration of love to God. Faith is a response of love to God.

Faith is our opportunity to grow. As we are, He loves us and He still wants us to grow. While we do not feel that we deserve the affects of our lives, we do deserve to <u>grow</u>. We deserve to experience God's glory through the trials and tribulations with which we are posed. Our trials are the builder of our testimonies. Our testimonies are the evidence of our faith. Our testimonies are for the other's whose lives we cross. Our testimonies require our transparency. This transparency represents growth, love, trust and freedom. This transparency represents our faith.

I knew I was growing as a Christian when I could imagine how I could share what God had done, when I could share what God had saved me from and when I considered what God has planned for me. Before the "ah-ha" moment, I was very private. I did not share my triumphs or my struggles with anyone. What I did not realize was that because I did not share the Lord's work in my life, I was blocking the blessings of myself and others. God could not use me the way He planned through all of my life's events if I would not share Him. However, I failed Him. I kept my lessons to myself. Now I do not keep them to myself. I share when appropriate. I am honest. I am open. I am compassionate. I am free. I am free when I share God's work in my life. My testimony is an exhibit of my faith.

What is your testimony? Are you telling those who cross your path who qualify to experience your testimony? Yes, I said qualify to experience your testimony. Qualify suggests that everyone cannot understand the testimony you may share. The person listening to your testimony has to be the right maturity level and for the right reasons to experience some of your testimony. Your testimony has power. This is not gossip that we repeat to each passerby. It has weight. God powers your testimony. He gives it energy and life. God gives it influence. What that means is that God uses your testimony to change, mature, influence and draw others close to Him. He uses His work in you to further His work in others.

Your testimony is an experience: God's experience. The persons who are listening or witnessing are having a God experience. They experience what God needs them to so that they can be in the position God needs them in so that He can deal with them as He has planned. It is not our job to do more or less. We are to share our testimony: at the right time, in the right place, to the correct persons. "How will I know?" You will be led to do so in such a compelling manner that you won't miss the opportunity.

The Faith Factor is a location where we want to live. However, it can be uncomfortable. What does the faith factor look like by God's definition? This is hard for me sometimes. So we will use Job as an example. Job had immense faith. He lost <u>everything</u>! EVERYTHING!!! His story is powerful. Job 1:8-22, 2:1-10. Satan asked God for permission to aggravate Job. God trusted Job so He permitted satan to deal with Job. God trusted Job! God had faith and confidence in Job's ability to remain faithful and committed to God.

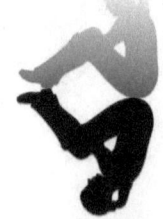

Job loses everything first. Job then has to manage his wife and friends. For this purpose, Job is naked and alone. Job could not depend on his wife. The wife suggested Job curse God. Job could not depend on his friends. They considered Job's position and situation to mean that God had abandoned Job. Job is a special man. Job uses this time, while he doesn't know it's temporary, to commune with God. satan was aware of the relationship between God and Job. satan insisted that God would never allow this type of activity to happen to Job. Yet God did allow it but told satan that there were limits to what he could do.

Job's response is the most important part. He gave all of himself to God. Consider how you have responded when "storms" have "come" to your life. Are you conditional? Do you make rash choices, bad decisions? God wants us to know how we will behave during a storm. Job does his part. Job was presented with several tests.

PASS or FAIL

Job's first test (1:14-15, 18-19) was his livestock and the children were killed. Job's reaction is highly unusual (v. 20 – 21). Job is heartbroken yet does not sin (v. 22). He does tear his clothing, shave his head and praise God. This test of Job's faith is customary as is our tests. Job passed the test: Job did not sin. God was proud of Job's reaction. Job remained connected with God. Job considered this a message from God and his response indicates that. Job acknowledges that ALL that he "owned" belongs to God. Job understands that the children and the livestock which he was assigned to as a steward still belong to God. Job reconciled since it all belongs to God, then God can have it back whatever He chooses. Job sets the following examples for us: (A) we do not own anything; (B) being a good steward does not

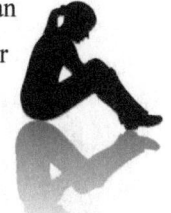

entitle us to anything; (C) we still praise God in what we have labeled as despair; (D) Job's humility is an extraordinary exhibit of Job's understanding of who God is; and, (E) Job didn't ask any questions.

As Job reconciles, God smiles. I can imagine God shaking His head when I determined that I am yet bold enough to question Him what He did provide for me. Our faith is the cornerstone of who we are. God still protected Job even though Job experienced pain. Job didn't argue, ask or critique God for his state of affairs. Job's faith was tested. Job's faith is exercised. The faith is determined by what we have passed or failed? We may fail our faith. We do often abandon our faith because faith requires trust. When I question God <u>and</u> sin, I say that I do not trust God.

When I trust God, my faith through my behavior is evident. I believe God for His sustainment of my soul, spirit, and my mind. God has kept me WHOLE through lots of events. My behavior is my attitude, my speech, my thoughts, my actions and my moods. Our behavior communicates our love via trust of God. When we doubt, we do not communicate love. When we doubt, we communicate fear. When you lack faith, we don't communicate love. Consider Job's behavior. Job realized that God owns it all, controls it all, distributes all, and designs at all. Job knows that he's just a manager. Job considers his relationship with God important and priority.

Job's second test was more intense because it was personal. satan struck Job with sores all over his body (2:7). It got personal! A personal attack is the worst type of attack. The personal attack is the most impacting, the most critical, and the biggest test. Well good news: Job passed test two. The question is whether we pass this personal test.

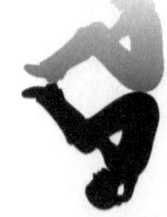

With these sores, Job communes even closer to God. He sits and scrapes the sores off of his skin. Job determines that he's going to take action to remove the scars. His wife walks up and says, "Curse God." He replies that she is foolish. She is foolish. Many of us are as well. What would we do as Job with our sores? Not probably behave the same. Certainly there is some anxiety as related to what to do. However, we are reminded that in his condition, he still did not sin (v. 10).

Job teaches us lessons throughout the chapter. His wife suggests that he also exercise behavior which would alienate us from God. Most of us do this daily anyway. Job teaches a profound lesson on faith and how it's measured. Faith is considered optional while God certainly does not treat us this way. Job demonstrates that faith is our life line. Job's faith is strong enough to share how to be faithful to others. Job explains that faith involves the good from God and the trouble. We want just the good. We would like to be excused from the trouble.

Job had three friends who supported him. Are we the kind of friends that would fast with our friend for seven days? They wept on his behalf. Are we the friend who will weep for another or do we abandon? Did the faith of the friends increase or was it enhanced through his experience? Did God get the glory from the encounter? What must they have thought about Job because they knew how Job loved God? How is their commitment level to God? Was that part of the reason for the experience to increase the commitment of the friends?

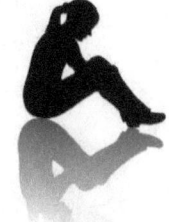

Let's explore how our faith can expand and increase based on the experience of others. When we see others' experiences, we should consider what does God want us to learn? How do we grow to the level of faith without seeing, living and experiencing different things? How can we apply Job's lessons to our lives?

Job does something interesting following the visits with his friends (Job 3). He curses the day he was born. He suggests that he should not have been born. He believes that his birth is a mistake. He suggests darkness over the days of his conception and birth. He begs to have not been born.

He faces his concept of his darkest hour. He perceives that he is not in need of being alive and that the world would be better if he had never been born.

Has your darkest hours sounded like that? Is that your call back to God? During your darkest hour, do you move closer to God? Faith does not happen in isolation. Faith grows in the presence of others. Faith requires the presence of others. It is not a private act. Faith requires the accountability of others. Faith is your accountability to others as well.

When Job addresses his wife about faith, he has to lead by example. He had to have an experience in order to share his faith with others. Others have to be challenged in some manner to make their faith come alive. Faith sharing is critical for the growth of us as a church. We all can afford some growth of our faith. God selects those of us who may not need the most growth but who He can depend on the most to operate with our faith and has the best opportunity to lead others to

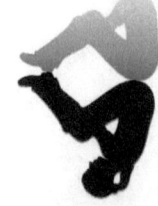

an increased faith. Faith is an exercise of mutual trust. God trusts us and we have to trust Him, only and ultimately. God selected Job because of the strong, STRONG mutual trust.

God sends us into the lives of others to share our faith and our testimony. As Christians, we are to encourage each other. We are to share our testimony, our fears, our pains and to confess our sins. Our safety should exist among other Christians.

Job's friend, Eliphaz, stood up for Job and encouraged him. Eliphaz shares powerful words of wisdom to Job. Eliphaz does not doubt God or His instructions. Eliphaz supports Job during his trials. Eliphaz speaks blessings in Job's life and his situation. Can we say that we have CONSISTENTLY done this? Do we instead speak death and demise and pain into the lives of others? Into our own lives? The power our tongues possess move mountains and creates love and peace that can become consumed with destruction and demise. Finally, Eliphaz offered wise advice. Job 5:8 reads, "But if it were I, I would appeal to God; I would lay my cause before Him." Eliphaz continues by explaining why this appeal is the best choice. For the next 28 verses, he explains the power of God as well as the benefits of a relationship with God. Eliphaz references some mighty events which bring a clear understanding of who God is and the extent of His sovereignty and mercy and grace. Eliphaz implores Job to exercise prudence as Job processes his situation. God has proven the God He is and does not give reason for doubt.

Job does not readily receive the encouragement of Eliphaz. This is too familiar. We do this: we reject the messenger who brings the

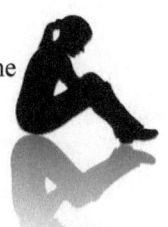

encouraging words yet we provide unconditional audience to those who speak doom into our lives.

Job argues for two chapters, six and seven, that God has forsaken him. Job suggests that he is burdened and weary, that he is being ignored by God. Job begs to know how he has wronged God: "show me where I have been wrong." Job 6:24b.

Job shares our attitude here when we only consider those who are wrong received this level of lesson. We defined what Job survives as punishment and pain, of which is only deserved by those who sin against God. Job does not see how he earned this punishment or deserves the situation. He asked in several ways how did he bring forth the wrath of God in this manner. The other factor which adds to Job's frustration is the fact that God is not answering him. Job feels that God should answer him. Upon command. Interestingly enough, we behave that same way. We take the creative license to take our time obeying and surrendering and submitting to God yet we want God to respond immediately, particularly since we do not "deserve" this activity anyway.

I ask myself often could I be Job. Could I do what God trusted Job with? When I consider Job, I usually think not so much. I do not think that I could have been Job but I have my own version of his story. At which point do I question God and what His intentions are? God uses us for His purposes. He does not owe us an explanation of His intentions.

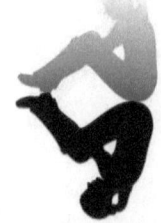

Job continues to plead for God's attention. Job 7:11 "therefore I will not restrain my mouth; I will speak in the anguish of my spirit; I will complain in the bitterness of my soul." Job would like to know what he needs to do next. He is begging for an explanation. He has given up the art of discretion, which many of us do when we call ourselves being frustrated with God. This season calls for patience with God because we are on His timing. God would like our honesty but with an immeasurable amount of respect. We are not strangers to "bitterness of my soul." There are at least a dozen counts where we could consider ourselves in that situation. God is gracious and forgiving and compassionate when these feelings surface.

Bildad, another friend of Job's, suggests Job's immediate repentance. Bildad asks Job four questions: (1) How long will you speak to God this way? (2) Do you know that your words are strong like the wind? (3) Does God overturn or ignore judgment? And (4) Or does God set justice aside for the sake of setting justice aside?

These four questions are designed to help Job understand that he was being disrespectful to God. Bildad opens chapter 8 with those same four questions. In verse five (8:5), Bildad persuades Job to earnestly seek God and plead with fervor to God. Bildad knew that God's wrath would or could deepen because Job's perceived disrespect. Bildad further concludes that God will not punish a blameless man (v. 20) or turn away from a righteous man to evildoers. He proceeds to mention that God will only fill us with laughter and give us reason to shout with joy. God further (v. 22) will protect us from our enemies.

As Bildad continues, it is important to mention that Bildad and Eliphaz probably never knew they would have such an opportunity to minister to Job in this manner. Our friends are very important. These are people who save us from ourselves when we are having trouble and in this case, when we are doubting God. Our friendship choices impact our faith. These choices have to be carefully decided. These friends have influence over the interpretations of what God wants, what God shares and what God expects. One wrong word from a "friend" could easily move us from where God intends for us. Friends can be distracting and they can also be a messenger from God to move us closer to God. The truest friends will draw us nearer to God. Bildad took a leap of faith of his own when he spoke to Job in reference to what he thought God wanted and deserved. Bildad took their friendship to a different level because it could have been seen as risky but Job received the words sent by God through Bildad.

Job responds (9:1) to Bildad that this is true. Job continues to speak to God's power and how that power affects the life of each of us. Job shares that God has powers above all other entities. Job thinks that he is not important to God. He states, "How then can I dispute with Him? How can I find words to argue with Him?" v. 14, and "Even if I summoned Him and He responded, I do not believe He would give me a hearing." V. 16. Job further declares that God will not seek to answer Job just because he is Job and he asked God. Job is examining his life from the lowest possible factor. Job does not realize that he is exercising the highest element of his faith.

Job had not previously been tested. This faith walk he embarks upon is unanticipated and lacked historical reference and that is how God planned it. Likewise, our faith calls for this purity. We cannot use historical reference to determine how to respond and should we respond with faith and which level or degree of faith. Each situation requires a different level of faith. Pure faith is always required. Some

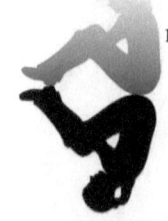

days require more faith than others. Your faith shows up differently daily. Faith is an act of obedience. Faith is an exercise of trust in God. Faith communicates to God that you believe that God has a plan (Jeremiah 29:11-12) and that He knows you well enough to know what you can handle (Psalm 139). He knows how you will respond in all situations. God promises us so much and loves us more than He promises. God promises that these situations are designed to move us beyond doubt and closer to Him.

As Job suggests further in chapter ten, God has made his obedience and goodness look cheap and stupid. He asks God if this was sport to God of favoring the wicked over his righteous life. If you have never challenged God in this manner, I ask His blessings for you right now. Many of us have this done that and much more. Verses four through seven, Job asks Him what kind of God are You. Job suggests that He's using the same filter humans are using since Job was chosen to suffer. Job contends that there are others who actually deserve this but are living without one blemish and no pain. Verse seven, Job acknowledges his claim and pronounces God's power yet again: "though you know that I am not guilty and that no one can rescue me from Your hand?" Job accepts the fact that God has him here and until God is done with the experience, here he will remain. Job continues to ask some extremely powerful questions about the relationship he has had with God. Job remarks in verse fifteen that "Even if I am innocent, I cannot lift my head, for I am full of shame and drowned in my own affliction." Job continues for seven more verses cursing his own birth and sentences himself to hell. Job considers his complete life unworthy of having been lived based on this experience.

YIELDED AND SUBMITTED

Measure your darkest hour(s) against Job's. When you consider the measure of loss and pain, have you been this low? I contend that if Job had not been accountable to his friends, wife and to God and a spiritually weaker man, he would have taken his own life. He gives that impression several times. It was not his life to take. He also keeps affirming that his life belongs to God (10:8-12). He asked Him again why did You bring me here if this was the outcome. The most powerful question was, "Are not my few days almost over?" verse 20. He assumes this "pain" is a sentence to death. Job has given up and hopelessness has set in his heart. He is not exercising any faith. He is operating on pain. Most of us have done this. He feels forsaken by God.

Zophar intervenes for Job as only a great friend can. For twenty verses, Zophar explains that God is not who you now knew Him as. Chapter 11, verse 6, Zophar explains that "true wisdom has two sides." Wisdom comes in the format of what we want to hear and what we don't want to be. Likewise, Zophar goes on to remind Job that "God has forgotten some of your sins." This begs the question: Did God forget because there were too many or because He made a choice to forget. We know that God makes a choice to forget. He's the same God who knows every strand of hair on my head; He can easily remember each of my sins. Zophar reminds Job that God has not forsaken him. God has Job firmly in His hands. Zophar suggests a renewal of the relationship (v. 13—14) so that our commitment to God is re-established.

Job finally admits that images have taken him captive (12:4). He is concerned that God has invalidated his witness to God's goodness amongst his friends and community. He continues by

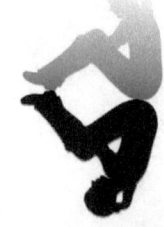

detailing God's wrath over others. He argues that He is not foolish. As he continues through chapter thirteen, he makes two very important statements (v. 3 and v. 24): I want to plead/argue my innocence to God and God why are You treating me as an enemy. Job desires answers from God. Questions we would have: (1) Why me Lord? (2) What have I done to deserve this Lord? (3) What can I do to make this stop Lord? (4) How long will this last Lord? (5) Why are You angry with me Lord? Job seeks an audience with God. He wants to know exactly when their relationship changed. Job continues through Chapter 14, noting God's powers and articulating God's options in how He manages us. Job compares us to a tree where the tree can grow again yet man cannot. Job offers powerful imagery as he explains his plight and prays for an audience with God.

Job listens to Eliphaz in Chapter15. Job responds in Chapter 16 with certainty, "I am alone." Job states that he would never have spoken to his friends the way they have to him. He makes this view of the wrath he is experiencing. His pain has been made great and shared publicly. This is the Source of further pain for us is when our "issues" are exposed to and subject to the judgment of others. Job scolds his friends for their words and lack of encouragement. In Chapter 16, verse 17, he shows himself as hopeful: "yet my hands have been free of violence and my prayer is pure." Job indicates that in spite all that I have gone through, I have not sinned. Job wants to know why this has happened to him. This question is very familiar to us, not matter how mature we are in Christ. This question is based on how severe the situation is and as a result how much He wants our faith to growth and how much He wants us to exhibit. Job continues in Chapter 17 this same sentiment: God has made a mockery of me and abandoned me.

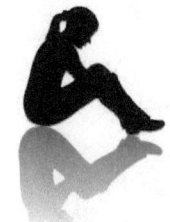

Verse 11 further exhibits his hopelessness: "My days are passed, my plans are shattered and so are the desires of my heart." In one set of events, the desired of his heart are gone!

Have you been there? Sure you have. What brought you out of that? What restored your faith? What made you stop your 'pity party'?

Bildad replies in Chapter 18 that Job is wicked because he is being punished. Bildad details that punishment for Job. He heaps coals of death on Job's dying spirit. Job banters with Bildad as he responds in Chapter 20. Job asks his friends how long will you speak negatively to me (v. 2) and attack me (v. 3). Job does not expect this attack and response from his friends. We expect them to encourage us and help us. Job considers the fact that he has been shunned and set aside by everyone that God has purposed this.

He makes several important points:

(1) He recognizes that God has moved him from "natural" influence. God has put him in an inaccessible place for others to reach him.
(2) He recognizes that God needs him inaccessible so that God can have Job's attention.
(3) Through all of that God is still my Redeemer—no matter what.
(4) At the end of this, I will see God.
(5) The pity of his friends will not sustain him.

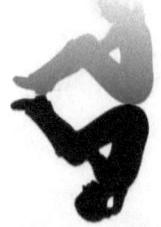

When he learns all of this, he resigns to the fact that he will be alone yet affirms that he will see God again, where in His presence, he will find peace.

Zophar reappears in Chapter 20 with more judgment for the wicked. He outlines the consequences for the wicked and seems to be sharing with Job that he has taken his fate into his own hands. Bildad and Zophar contend that Job brought this on himself and his "speeches" demanding God's answers and attention are deepening and intensifying the wrath of God.

From Chapters 21-37, for 438 scriptures, the five of them, including Elihu, banter back and forth about God, Job's sins, their judgment of Job and their thoughts and recommendations.

Job clarifies, in Chapter 21, that part of his argument is that "people who do not love God do not bear this level of pain nor endure this turmoil." "Why should a righteous man such as myself have so much agony, pain, ridicule and disconnect from God?" Job actually implies that the wicked never see the repayment for their evil (v. 19—21). Job still thinks the friends should be offering consolation but they are not.

Eliphaz accuses Job of ignoring the work of God. From verses 4 to 9 of Chapter 22, Eliphaz states that Job took clothing from man, denied water to the weary, denied food to the hungry and sent widows away with nothing to name a few of Job's sins. Eliphaz states that these oversights and the exact cause Job's struggle (v. 10—11). Eliphaz accuses Job of walking in wickedness (v. 23) and continuing to ignore the teachings of God.

Job's response in Chapter 23 is that he is looking for God to share his bitterness. Job shares that he is terrified of God because of His power and the ability to complete "many such plans he still has in store" v. 14b. He admits his fear but is determined not to be silent (v. 16—17). Job's interested in justice. He points out the sins of each dark character of which he can thrive. Job questions why they are allowed to continue such indiscretions without penalty. He argues that he has done nothing as bad as they even if his childhood sins are remembered.

In Chapter 25, Bildad responds with similar responses as he previously offered. In Chapter 26, Job continues forward with more questions about God's judgment and who is getting away with all the sins of which he speaks. Job is exercising shallow judgment though. He doesn't have enough information to make that assumption. At any rate, he compares his life to the life of others which is always dangerous. What God does for and to others has no bearing on what we receive or how He manages us. God treats us as He decides.

God expects our faith to transcend this level where we consider what God does for others in comparison to what He does for us. Our faith requires purpose. Faith is required for a powerful and an outstanding walk with God. Job does do something great that the rest needs to note: Job seeks God fervently. Job does not give up on finding and talking to God. Seeking God requires a deep and authentic faith. While Job is outwardly focused on what appears to his friends as crazy and spiritually suicidal, he is inwardly focused on trying to figure out how he went wrong in God's eyes. Seeking God's favor requires faith. Do we have that measure of faith? Job wants God's justice. He feels that he has lived a life which deserves God's favor and little or no

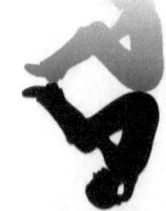

punishment at all. He feels that he has worked hard for that reward. Chapter 27:6 reads "I will maintain my righteousness and never let go of it; my conscience will not reproach me as long as I live." I cannot always stand on integrity and the quality of my conscience. I deserve those punishments and I am the recipient of His mercy, grace and forgiveness. So are you. Remember that God does whatever He desires. He disciplines us as He decides regardless of what we desire or think.

    Job professes some profound statements in Chapter 28. Faith is fluid. Job shares the wisdom for which he was previously known. Job had moved into an academic, an almost worldly attitude, and now he was returning to a spiritual disposition, a retreat attitude. We now see Job discuss the wonders of God. Job's detailed description of the creation and location of natural resources which speaks to God's awesome planning and thought process. Job shares the location of the world's most treasured natural resources turned assets, then asks comparatively. "But where can wisdom be found? Where does understanding dwell? Man does not comprehend its worth; it cannot be found in the land of the living," (v. 12—13). Job continues to compare the pricelessness to the value of those same precious and highly sought commodities. He further illuminates that this wisdom and understanding is only known by God (v. 23). Job confirms that God is the author of all wisdom. To acquire this God created wisdom, seeking God is required and faith is the bridegroom. Verse 28 clearly reminds us, confirming that Job has his wits about him. "And he said to man, "The fear of the Lord—that is wisdom, and to shun evil is understanding,"" Job is seeking God and will continue to do so. Faith keeps him seeking God and not quitting until He finds Him.

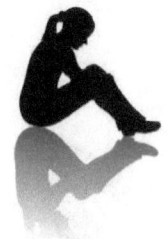

Job reminisces on who he was before this catastrophe. He recalls how people responded to him. He remarks on the impact he had on the community. He notes his high position among the people and the authority he enjoyed and exercised. Does any of that sound familiar to you? Job never anticipated this situation of total loss. Because of his position, authority, wisdom, and other privileges, he never thought that this would happen. He was in the will of God enjoying all of His favor. Job took God's favor seriously and did not take advantage. For this reason, he finds these new circumstances unreasonable as well as overwhelming. The respect and regard others had for Job was based on the position Job has given. When God "afflicts" him, all of this passes, (30:11). In Chapter 30, he shares how they now they behave. This is truly how we uplift people because of stuff rather than who they are inside and their calling. Our calling is not attached to our material belongings. He created the voice, mind, heart and esteem to serve Him and His regardless of our financial state and material possessions. We do this out of faith. We serve others because we are called. Our faith will sustain the calling and support our assignment. Faith keeps us during the times we don't see the value of our contribution.

Job declares in 30:21 that God has "turned on him ruthlessly." Job's perception and our similar ones unravel our faith. Job spends the next ten verses continuing to build his defense for why he is undeserving of God's "wrath." For the forty verses of Chapter 31, Job declares his innocence and contends he should be held blameless. He almost mocks God with an ultimatum of presenting an indictment against him (v. 35). Surely a bold move by Job. Wise—not so sure. The only glimmer of hope rests with Job's ability to recount his living and

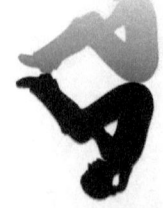

how he craved to please God. Faith is required to crave God at that level, through that pain, throughout that situation and circumstances.

In the next five chapters, 32—37, Elihu speaks to Job. Job does not respond. Elihu is the youngest of the four friend—advisors. He speaks after the others out of respect and now his anger has sparked the need to share. Wisdom is not given based on age. Elihu spends 22 verses explaining that the spirit within compels him to speak, that the other three have not answered Job's argument and setting the stage for some much needed wisdom. Elihu uses Chapter 33 to establish his credentials to be able to share his knowledge and information. Within those 33 verses of Chapter 33, Elihu asks Job to carefully reconsider what he has said to God. Elihu has challenged the righteous picture that Job has pointed for himself. Elihu further notes that Job has tried to equate himself to God. Elihu cautions Job to consider the whole image of God—which Job has neglected in his previous presentations, according to Elihu. Elihu offers to teach Job wisdom (v. 33).

In Chapter 34, Elihu addresses more of Job's righteous claims. Elihu contradicts each one. Elihu shares a different picture of God, the cause of his wrath, and our response to God, whether anger, or mercy. Elihu suggests that "Job's words lack wisdom" (v. 35). Elihu considers 'to his sin he adds rebellion' and 'he multiplies his word against God' (v. 37). Chapter 35, for 16 verses, Elihu encourages Job to consider God and what He wants and expects. Elihu encourages us to consider carefully your approach to God and what God may think of us and our behavior. Elihu suggests that Job has a general misunderstanding of God and His ways. Elihu implies that this misunderstanding extends to us as well.

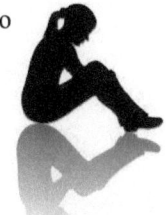

YIELDED AND SUBMITTED

Elihu teaches praise in Chapter 36, for 33 verses. Elihu shares considerable details about God which had been left unmentioned by the other four men before. Elihu reminds that the knowledge of God is made known to us by God, not by ourselves. Elihu reminds Job that God's care is extensive: "Indeed He would have brought you out of dire distress, into a broad place where these is not restraint and what is set on your table would be full of richness" (v. 16).

Elihu's bold and strong approach is profound in that he has taken a non-negotiable stance because he feels led and is operating on faith which God will honor. God is carefully considering these 36 chapters because He permitted the events, which has led them to these conversations. Elihu has spoken freely and objectively with passion. His wisdom will be considered by God.

Elihu closes his discourse in Chapter 37 without an opportunity for a single interruption from Job or the others, yet with an attitude of zeal and worship. Elihu inspires and challenges a new attitude toward God. Elihu expressed pure adoration for God's work and His abilities and His wonders. Elihu influences amazement at God and all that He is and all that He does. Elihu reminds us to adjust our attitude toward God.

For the next four chapters, God speaks. God asks Job forty-two questions in Chapter 38. God asks Job in quite the frustrated tone is Job more than He, with these 42 questions in 41 verses. God asks Job some specific questions which speak to and confirm the ultimate power of God, of which Job obviously needed to be reminded.

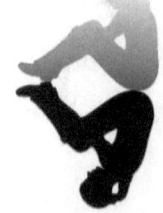

God gave him such a detailed description of what he did not know. God starts with the Earth's foundation (v. 4—7) with an adamant tone of how dare you question Me about what I am doing. God expounds on controlling the waves and the boundaries of the sea (v. 11). God extends His lesson by deepening our understanding of the finest of details: "Have you ever given orders to the morning" (v. 12). God shares with Job, and by extension us, that our global thoughts have failed and lacks substance. The other factor is that would the morning even listening to us, even if He bestowed powers to us to order the morning to start? He knows that would not be the case, which further stimulates His fury at Job because of his attitude. One of the most profound exhibits of God's authority is when God asks if Job could change a wasteland to grassyfield (v. 25—27). "Does the rain have a father? Who gives birth to the drops of dew? (v. 29)." This is so transparent and detailed for the consideration of God. In verse 35, God asks a question: "Do the lightning bolts report to you, here we are?" God reinforces that we have wisdom and understanding because of Him. God reminds Job of some pivotal details which speak volumes of His profound power.

God opens Chapter 39 sharing that He knows when each of us gives birth and He is present for each birth. God shares that He is all-knowing and well-planned and the gift-giver of life. We are foolish when we are not realizing that God is God. He knows what exact time we will birth the offspring we have been blessed to carry. He blesses the birth and ends the birth pains. God ends Chapter 39 asking Job is the eagle at Job's command and does it seek Job for food.

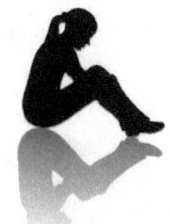

God invites Job to speak in Chapter 40: "Let Him who accuses God answer Him!" Job answers God ever so wisely. "I am so unworthy—how can I reply to you?" (v. 2). Job repeats that he is unworthy to speak and reply to God. God starts again in verse six with more questions, but the most important question in verse eight, "Would you discredit My justice? Would you condemn Me to justify yourself?" God continues to ask Job companion questions: one of which was God's arms comparable to Job's or was the voice of God like Job's? God wants us to understand that He is not like us. He does God-sized projects with God-sized visions and God protects those who serve Him diligently. God presents Himself with the facts of what He has done consistently to all of us at all times. God has accurately articulates that He has been there with each milestone and mistake and victory. He has withheld nothing from us. He has been the strength, peace, crafter, author, and orchestrator of the finest details of our lives.

Chapter 41 continues to detail God's works. God asks 'can or will' for several verses and Job remains quiet. Verse 10 reads: "No one is fierce enough to rouse him. Who then is able to stand against Me?" As a Christian, I have no ability to stand against God. I advise you to reconsider before you use this approach. When you are hurt or angry enough to consider that approach, you may want to confess your heart to God such that God may have time to show you what God is doing in your life. This is an opportunity for extravagant faith with God's leadership. The process from fear, frustration, and pain to joy, peace, and love. Faith is required to endure our percentage of misfortune. What happens to us is for our good. Faith is required to understand how that applies.

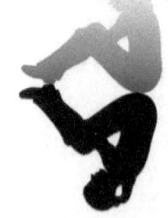

Job had proposed quitting. He wanted to die. He asked to be relieved of his life. God never planned that so that request and suggestion was ignored and denied. Did God anticipate Job's response? I am not sure that what He expected from Job but what Job actually did offended God. Our job is not to offend God. Our actions should not offend God. Our lack of faith also offends God.

Verse 11 of Chapter 41 reads, "Everything under heaven belongs to Me," reinforces that God is the owner and we are simply the managers. He does not owe us anything! Once we really understand that our journey is so much easier. Because of His blessings and coverings, we become Proud. I am accustomed to being cared for by God. I am accustomed to having everything God has given so when I want something, I am not accustomed to no. He is King over me even when I am proud (verse 34). God does not honor pride, yet He does not abandon or cast us out without giving us an opportunity to repent of that pride.

Job responds to God in Chapter 42 in an humble fashion which submits to God his apologies for being out of line. Job admits his ignorance (verse 3) of "things too wonderful for me to know." Job witnesses to the power of God through seeing Him rather than just hearing Him. Job confesses that he despises himself and repents without condition. Job prepares to accept WHATEVER God issues for him. Job is not expecting anything from God. Job does not ask God for ANYTHING.

God praises Job and reprimands his friends for their words and messages about God. God instructs them to submit a sacrifice to God

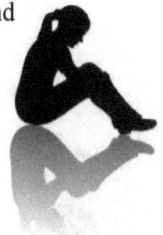

through the very one they reprimanded, Job. God guides them to restitution through Job's prayers (verses 7—9).

God does several things after the reprimand of Job's friends. God restores Job's wealth by twice his previous amount, Job's community position and influence and leadership. Job is reunited with all of his family, friends, acquaintances and with zeal they visited with him, bringing the gift of silver and a gold ring (verses 10—11).

Further, God replaced and increased Job's flock exponentially. The best portion of Job's restoration was the blessing of ten children. In a time when women are overlooked for inheritances, Job shared his wealth equally amongst his children without gender discrimination.

Job lived one hundred forty years so for four generations, his children and grand-children experienced God's favor through Job, as well as hear and experience his faith and testimony.

Job creates a picture for us of faith and genuine commitment to God for the service of God. Job claimed several lessons during this time frame which he passes on to us.

Job's wife thought he had earned his way from trouble. This is not possible. God will test us under whatever circumstances He deems necessary. God wants to know what He can trust us with. The only way to know is to be tested through storms. Our storms develop within us a testimony which God has created, designed and developed to be told and transmitted to certain audiences at certain times to bring glory to God, Himself. This pre-determined and pre-destined "trouble" distances us from the average Christian.

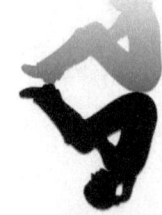

THE FAITH FACTOR

Job is a trusted servant of God. God had to remind Job as well as others of His sovereignty and His glory. While He reminds Job, He reminds that He is in charge of everything; full power and dominion rests completely with Him.

Those destined for greatness can count on some storms. God does not allow us to see the fruits without some labor. He needs us to exhibit our maturity to handle the gifts we are about to receive. The people we admire and aspire to be, have a testimony, a story on how they arrived to this point and how that helped them to reach this level. God has to know that a new level will not separate us from Him. God is selfish and jealous. He is not going to elevate us in such a manner or increase us where we will forget the God we serve, adore and worship.

Faith is required to please God. When this series of events started, Job was not excited but understood that his fate was with God. He would not curse or sin against God. God wants us to have faith that He has our best interest in mind. Faith that He has a fully executable plan where He will be glorified at the end and during. Faith where He will sustain us while we are here in the midst. Faith that He hears us, and answers our prayers. Finally we need enough faith to share our testimony and dilemmas with others. Faith is cultured among believers and those we are growing in faith. Faith is evidence of things hoped for but yet seen. Job has grown the faith of the people around him.

Questions you have to answer about your faith:

- Am I faithful?
- What grows my faith?
- What causes my faith to falter or fail?

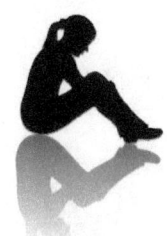

- Do I know when my faith is about to fail?
- Do I know why my faith is being tested?
- Do I know what to do with my faith?
- Do I know what God needs from me?
- Do I know who to share my faith with?
- What do I do when my faith is about to fail?
- Does my faith demonstrate my love for God?
- Do others know the measure of my faith?
- Do others get nervous when I go through storms?
- Do others know how much I trust God?
- Do I realize that my faith is on display for others to grow?
- Does the measure of my faith honor God?
- Does the faith I have please God?
- What do I gain when God is pleased with my faith?

On a journey dedicated to God, your faith has already been tested, stretched, reshaped and reinvested. God is faithful and we should be likewise. God is the author of the journey. This is His journey. He requires our faith. Faith is parallel to His calling on your life. Your life will not be great without faith. Faith comes with experiences which cause your faith to expand. God never blamed satan. satan never reappears. This building of faith only involved you and God. The life He makes for us is based on the measure of our faith.

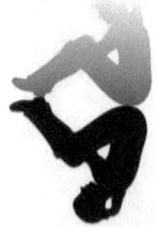

The Fear Factor

Fear of man will prove to be a snare,
But whoever trusts in the Lord is kept safe.

Proverbs 29:25
New International Version (NIV)

For God did not give us a spirit of timidity, but a spirit of power, of love and self-discipline.

2 Timothy 1:7
New International Version (NIV)

Fear has been acronymed as false evidence appearing real. What is your definition of fear? How long have you had that definition? How have you lived through and around that fear?

Webster defines fear as an unpleasant often strong emotion caused by anticipation or awareness of danger. Webster also defines fear as a reverential awe of God.

There are said to be 365 appearances of the word fear in the Bible. This would include passages which instruct us not to fear.

Gage's theory of fear is often optional and fear is also subjective. We are not fearful of the same things. There are hundreds of phobias. All fear, except for the fear of God, is only in our minds. I fear snakes. I do not like snakes. I do not want to see them in any format: the zoo, the television, the movies, or anywhere. The fear is based on lack of knowledge. Fear is a conscious decision not to admit risk. Let's examine what really creates fear: success, failure, judgment, accountability, and any other elements which require change and discomfort and risk.

The fear of the Lord is not optional rather required. The "reverential awe of God" is a love relationship with God. This reverence to God is a relationship building period. Why do we revere God? Why should we revere God? Why do not we revere God? God deserves our reverence. When I say the word awesome, it is not the same as a basketball game or sale at the mall as when I refer to God. God is not equal to the car I drive or the purse I carry or the food I eat. I cannot use the same words or expressions when I refer to and speak of and speak to God.

Reverence includes our thoughts, words and behavior. Reverence is in response to what we know, experience, share and can testify about God, Jesus Christ and the Holy Spirit. The reverence we express happens in a number of mediums: thoughts, words and behavior.

Reverent thoughts of God include the thoughts we share about God and our meditative thoughts. Reverent thoughts prove to God that we are focused on Him. Reverent thoughts remind us that God is sovereign. God reads our minds and knows what we are thinking so consider that we need to keep that space as pure as possible. When I consider the unworthy thoughts which pass by my mind on a daily basis, it is hard to comprehend that He would still want to occupy the same space with me. That is just the thoughts which pass by, but what about the thoughts which stay, then the ones on which I act, and then I think some thoughts repeatedly act on them and never let them escape. This is not pleasing to God. While I am not reverent, He forgives me,

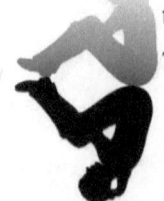

still has plans for me, still gives me life, still gives me strength, still gives me vision, still gives me passion and on and on. God is still focused on me and my needs and my gifts. Through all of that I do and do not revere Him. Through my sin: past, present and future.

Reverence is required. God does not need our relationship. Relationship and reverence are a pair. We need God! In that relationship, we need to revere God. Reverence costs! It costs our attention to God. It costs you to understanding why we revere God. It costs us to seek purity. It costs to separate from those who keep us away from God and godliness. It costs us to be transparent before God. It costs us honesty. It costs us the study of Him and His word. It requires us to deny ourselves in order to follow Him (Luke 9:23).

God is sovereign which is defined as having supreme rank, power, or authority. Likewise sovereign is defined as supreme, preeminent, indisputable, excellence, and in the greatest degree, utmost or extreme. God is above all of our stuff and nonsense and foolishness and dramatics. God does not think like us (Isaiah 55:8) nor does He behave like us. Understanding His sovereignty may take a while but the start of it is to understand He exists on a higher plane that what our finite minds, hearts, souls and methods can understand. Fear of God demonstrates the understanding that at least we are on our way to a meaningful relationship.

In this text, I will extend God to include Jesus Christ and the Holy Spirit. Fear of Them would be inclusive based on reverence and relationship. Jesus Christ earned our reverence and respect because He lived among us for 33 years without sin and was tempted just as we are.

YIELDED AND SUBMITTED

The Holy Spirit moves within our lives to stand in the gap for us on all of our issues. The Holy Spirit is a gift from God and Jesus Christ. Again understand the Holy Spirit is based on relationship. Waiting to hear from the Holy Spirit is part of building the relationship you need to be aligned with the Holy Spirit. The reverence required to understand both Jesus Christ and the Holy Spirit requires your heart and mind and soul.

Our reverence should lead to a unique peace where worry and fear does not exist. However, this is not always the case. Jesus offers us rest from burdens and weariness (Matthew 11:25—30) for those who come to Him. Matthew 11:28 reads, "Come to me, all you who are weary and burdened, and I will give you rest." Jesus offers His love through many means. This method would be thoughts among the top five demonstrations of his love. Rest for the weary and burdened is a consistent, non-conditional offer to all of us. When I say that it is non-conditional, you may challenge my interpretation because it reads "Come . . . And I will." Yes, we have to do something first before He gives us our desired rest. You have to Come to Jesus. That is an action rather than condition. Taking action should be your natural reaction.

Fear of God, as exhibited throughout the Bible, is critical. My favorite people in the Bible have a fear and reverence of God which serves as an example to us to understand how important it is for us to revere Him. To name a few and in no particular order: Esther, Ruth, Naomi, David, Joseph, Paul, John the Baptist, Mary, Noah and Job. While just as notable, Samuel and Solomon bring an upgraded definition to reverent and the reward for such.

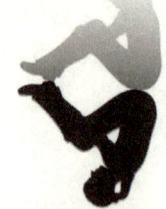

Each of them revered God through word, deed or both. Let's ask spend some time examining their reverence and the outcome of that fear of God. Their stories are unique but equally as instructional. Psalm 103:11 and 13 reads: "For as high as the Heavens are above the Earth, so great is His loving kindness toward those who fear Him. [13] Just as a father has compassion on his children, so the Lord has compassion on those who fear Him."

A Man After God's Own Heart

These words were authored by David so let us start with him and he is fear of God. David has a trust and a fear for God which stands out of all Bible persons, except One, as an overwhelming example of fear of God and its costs and its benefits.

David was chosen at an early age to be king of Israel. As a result of this election, David received many privileges and much favor from God. Fear of God includes obedience to God. David could have killed King Saul, his predecessor, three times. However, it was not in God's plan for David to strike Saul. David did send Saul a message each time though through his actions. In one instance, he cut Saul's cloak and left the piece for Saul to see. As you may understand that in order to get to the King in those days, there was a lot required—skill, negotiation and favor.

When David assumed the throne as king, he fought many wars, seen many victories and enjoyed the weight of God's favor. Because of his fear of God, he was promised the opportunity to erect the temple. However there was a significant time when David sinned but did not seek God for repentance. That cost David the opportunity to build the original temple God promised. David took a moment to be selfish which demonstrated his lack of respect for God.

David's most serious offense was when he starts to count his troops (2 Samuel 24). David stops trusting God and begins to fear men. God was angry at this act. David repented after he realized that he had acted inappropriately. David broke God's heart. God punished David through Israel for three days, putting to death 70,000 people and was going to kill more but God felt compassion for David's repentance and his request for mercy and stopped the plague. David's lack of fear of God cost the lives of others—not his own.

In a widespread of studies, David is labeled and named, "A Man After God's Own Heart." With such a label, one might ask how does a man with such a weighty name doubt God or question God or have a lack of fear of God. I have asked that question: How is it that how could such a highly favored man have such a lack of judgment or a such a severe lapse of judgment? How did David make such a bad decision? This teaches us that we must consider our weaknesses in our lives: do not forsake the fear of the Lord. Maybe because this is hard but the fear of the Lord is required and He will help us if we ask.

Reverence for God is shared with others. Your reverence can be contagious and should be. This reverence is not announced. It is simply experienced. How you respect God and fear Him is evident in all ways your speech, your tone, your behavior, your dress, your attitude, and your praise and worship.

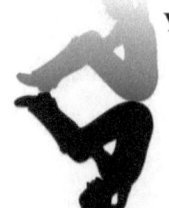

Your Speech

When you share your reverence through your speech, you are speaking with wisdom and kindness and care. This also means we abandon foul language. Our language cannot represent God and be foul. Likewise, we cannot belittle or berate or put down others. We do not trade insults. We speak prayerfully and carefully as to not embarrass God. Our speech has power to encourage and discourage, create life and sentence others to death, decipher and discerning, discriminating and discovering; our speech forces change—whether positive or negative.

I personally, and if you are honest, you do too, have the power to motivate others to be outstanding and successful. I can motivate you out of depression, hopelessness, brokenness, and self-destruction. This is the power of the tongue. Conversely, I can cause that same depression, hopelessness, brokenness, and self-destruction. As Christian woman, we are to uplift each other. We are designed to lift each other. We are someone's Ruth and we are someone's Naomi. There is no difference between us and a non—Christian if we our words do not sound different. We have to guard our mouths and our intentions. Because of our reverence, we should speak that reverence before others through our words and delivery thereof.

Your Tone

I have to be careful with my tone. When I speak, I have to ask myself if I sound like I am loving and kind and patient. I have to measure whether when I speak my tone is uplifting and encouraging rather than condescending and rude. Tone constitutes 38% of what makes up a conversation. So what does my tone say to others about me? So my tone is important to share with others. Likewise tone could change my message and change the weight of my message. Furthermore translates the message to others with passion and conviction rather than with condemnation and ridicule. God allowed me some places so that I can share my walk with others in a way which moves others closer and closer to God according to His will.

Tone is easily controlled by taking time your time to speak and consider how your voice will sound as it leaves your lips. I must practice this almost each time I speak. My tone will make all the difference in the world for whether or not it is received well or not. My tone can communicate how I consider and perceive the person, the topic and how I respect that relationship. My tone will share whether I am trying to be old, foster and create this relationship or if I am going to disrupt, destruct, and dissolve an unformed relationship. My tone will charge with love or challenge and create adversity.

A tone full of love and compassion and grace is what we should have. The recipient and audience will benefit from that seasoned tone. What we say is so important that we need them to receive what we need them to receive. The tone of the love confirms our reverence for God. There is nothing like wondering if "she" is a Christian. You asked that question because she just used foul and mean language to the sales clerk. Loudly. She is being rude and hurtful. She is a Christian to answer your question. She is out of order. She is operating out of the realm of reverence. She is not acting out of reverence for God. Her behavior is irreverent.

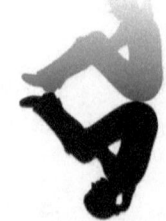

How does she fix this? How is this solved? How can she be assisted to behave reverently? Everyone has a bad day the difference is how we handled it. By the way, I have become more well—behaved since then. I do get angry and selectively so. I do get frustrated.

Your Behavior

One day, I was REALLY sharing with someone the fullness of my irritation with her poor customer service. I let her know how her skill set was unacceptable and less than adequate. I went on and on. At a point I realized that I was being harmful. I was no longer being the teacher-coach for which I am known. I was being outrageous. I had sinned. I treated her less than the child of God she is. Oh my God! When I realized my ultimate error and sin treating her like she was less than . . . me, I immediately stopped. I had embarrassed God. What should have been a coaching opportunity had become a bashing session. As the mature, experienced, post-retail manager, Christian, coach, gifted as preacher, teacher, and leader, I should have NEVER done that. I am designed to operate because of love, with love, and based on love. When I speak, I should say EVERYTHING with the love of God. When I cannot speak with that love God prescribes and desires, then I should refrain from speaking.

My behavior embarrassed God. God sent me in that space in her presence at that time for a specific purpose. I may have been called to witness or invite her to church or to hear her troubles and minister to her. I BLEW IT. I will never have that same opportunity again. I missed an opportunity to be trusted by God. I acted irreverently. God planned to use me to add to and strengthen His kingdom and I was distracted by my selfishness.

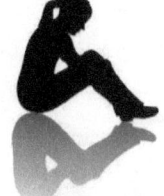

I made another error too: I broke her spirit. I damaged the spirit and possibly the self-esteem of another human being, specifically a woman. That is among the highest offenses. In our society, despite worldly objectives to decrease the spiritual influence, I strive not to put down or damage another woman. Women are harsh and hurtful and poisonous to each other. We should not be its way. God put us on this earth for certain reasons. One of those reasons is for us to mentor to one another (Titus 2:3-5). We cannot continue to treat each other in this foul, un-loving manner, and still expect the blessings of Christ. We are dainty creatures. We are fragile spirits. God protects us from the wrong persons entering our space. God cannot afford for us to fall into the wrong hands.

Your Spirit

A broken spirit requires healing. Healing requires time. Time requires commitment. Commitment produces desire. Desire produces motivation. All needed to completely and properly heal. Healing requires faith. You have to believe you will be healed. Mark 5:24-34 explains the statements I just made.

Reverence and fear of the Lord requires us to uplift others and behave accordingly. Out of my personal relationship with God which includes my fear of Him, I should be motivated to love others. Because of me is how He shows His love for others. So if I am misbehaving, I am not giving God's love away. However if I am behaving and following God's instructions, then I can enhance her self-esteem and improve her self-worth. I can exhibit my reverence and fear of God through loving others unselfishly. How I behave is critical to God's kingdom. There is the statement which is "We are the only, Jesus some people will ever see." This means that we are some persons only opportunity to be introduced to God and Jesus. We have to behave in a manner that does not take others away from God but drive them to God. One additional aspect of what I realized about my poor and possible pretentious behavior is that as a woman we don't need anything else to lower our self-esteem. If you are anything like me, you beat yourself up pretty good, so I don't need any help lowering my self-esteem.

As a disciple of Christ, and we all are, we are to edify others. Jesus describes in John, particularly John 14:34-35, "A new command I give you: love one another. As I have loved you, so you must love one another. [35] By this all men will know you are my disciples, if you love one another."

"And you call yourself a Christian!" Can this be said about us sometimes? Absolutely, our growth in Christ means that we have fewer of these occasions. God knows that we fear Him when we behave as a representative of Him.

Your Dress

For most of this chapter you have witnessed my testimony, so this will be different—a little. I dress conservatively. I wear longer skirts and looser pants. I do not like to call attention to my body. I have an average sized body. I could lose a few pounds and be in a bit better shape. So my next comments are based on observations which I consider critical to us as women.

I am a firm believer that the length of our skirts is relative to our self-esteem level. "Rev. Onedia, why would you say that? They have nothing to do with each other." Yes, they do. We use clothing to get the attention of others. We use our clothing to draw attention to ourselves because we crave attention and love. Our clothes get us that uplift. Most of us dress how we feel. I am going to challenge you today to lengthen your skirts, loosen your clothing, and dress well daily.

Self image is a hard to maintain project. It requires time, effort and self-esteem. They increase with mutual relativity. Your image is important because you represent God. I realize that is highly debatable, however, I feel that the short skirt does not please God. The short skirt requires more discipline with seating, standing, and all other movements. Likewise, the short skirt may introduce possible sin into the equation. Sin which you may be able to avoid with a longer skirt. What are we really saying with a longer skirt? I venture to say that we are promoting maturity, seriousness, and "lust-lack" attractiveness. I want a man who sees me to consider the words which come out of my mouth serious and worthy. I cannot afford for him to be standing there thinking of ways to create opportunities for me to sin. Likewise my dress should not influence that behavior. We may not have that intention because our intention was just get him to say 'hi' and make them jealous. I challenge us to decide on someone we respect to be that "judge" of our dress. There are ladies who I love and respect who would be concerned about my attire if it were too tight and too short. My dress illuminates my character. My dress shares my personality. My dress communicates my intentions.

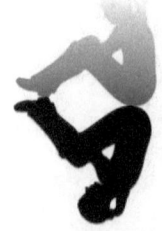

When I wear something questionable, it is so uncomfortable that I do not have a good time. I am conscious of the eyes of others. I have taught teenagers, a whole high school of them. Their self-esteem is driven by who likes them, who likes what they wear, what they have, and the electronics they carry. Notice I did not say how smart or what their grades are or how early they turned in their homework. At some point we have to transition to our self-esteem being driven by the factors which God considers important.

I preached a sermon entitled "Does She Know that He Loves Her" with text referencing Ephesians 3:14—21. This text describes the definition of God's love for us. This is possibly the third most important love scripture which defines for us God's love for us. This sermon was important because we create self-issues by allowing others to define who we are through less than satisfactory means. It is a challenge to understand how love is defined, created, and sustained: God. Others love us for a lot of conditional reasons. If you don't believe, change those superficial things and monitor the response(s).

If he knows me and finds me genuinely attractive, then he will be attracted to me while wearing a graduation robe. My body should not be the most attractive aspect about me.

With that said let's work on the other aspects of ourselves. Your mind, heart, intellect, creativity and whatever else is a part of you which should be attractive to you, not others, because God made you and ALL of your details.

There was a time when my ex-husband had really taken my self-esteem down. He would not talk to me. He did not compliment me.

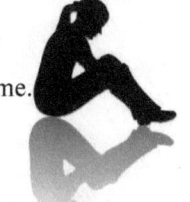

He did not find me attractive. He did not make me feel good. He did not make love to me. I kept asking him, begging him. One day God tapped me on the heart and spoke to me saying, "I love you! That's all that matters. You live to love, please, glorify and worship me. Not that husband, not those children. Just Me!" I got up from my pity party and my crying sessions and I prayed that God would show me what to do. I dusted the goal sheet off that I had accumulated over the years but never even started to pursue. When God spoke those words to me, I immediately knew I could hold my head up again. I still wanted him to talk to me but I was on my way to healing from brokenness.

God used the time after that to sharpen my mind. I returned to school and earned my Masters in Business Administration and Masters in Education. I started working on my Masters in Christian Education and my doctorate in Business. He blessed me to publish six additional books, totaling eight published. God enhanced our relationship. God moved me where He wanted me. God will send me to someone wonderful who thinks highly of what God does through me. I am able to share how God has moved in my life so that I can help other girls and women through several programs He has started through me.

So ask yourself, 'What does God want me to do? What has He called me to do? What have I not done on my "list" which God put in me to do?' The time which the answers to these questions require should consume enough time so that any negative, non-supportive, and short-skirt audiences can be applicably ignored.

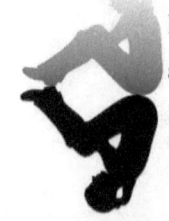

When God is first, the skirts will come down, the clothes will loosen and the self-esteem will improve, the self-worth will increase and the self-image will reflect that of our Maker. The people who you will attract will be different as well. How you respond to all people will change—remember the tone, speech and behavior discussions we just had. I started this discussion about dress with a disclaimer because I do not have any "short" dress stories. I have low-esteem stories. When I am out of close relationship with God, when I have moved out of His reach, I have deeply low self-esteem and extreme self-doubt. If I know this is the result, why move away from God?

The answer is our comfort ability. We get comfortable with our blessings, forgetting the Source and losing our focus. Some people call it "reading your own press" or "believing your own hype." The better life is going, the closer we should move toward God. I mentioned earlier that David had sinned. David's sin was sex with Bathsheba and the murder of her husband. David was being greedy and had coveted another man's wife. Because they had sex, she became pregnant. David covered the pregnancy by bringing her husband home from war in hopes that the couple would have intercourse then be able to pass the baby off as the husband's. That plan failed. The next step was that he murdered the husband, and married Bathsheba.

In this context, I have some questions. First, why didn't Bathsheba say no? Well it's the same reason we say yes when we should say no. Between jeopardized self-esteem and loneliness, Bathsheba consented. Bathsheba's skirt was short. She attracted someone to her when that should not have happened.

Secondly, Bathsheba could have confessed. Why didn't she? We never hear about her feelings or thoughts about what happened. But she could not confess because she consented. Let us consider some possibilities of her confession. Did she want to stay with David? Of course, she did. She consented. Could she have said no to the king? Maybe and maybe not. The point is that there were two responsible people and we only know how God held David responsible.

We are emotional beings. We respond to the events with the emotional response which is at any level hard to comprehend. Bathsheba liked the attention. She liked being summoned by the king. Being with the king had obvious benefits and he had catered to her emotional needs.

Those emotional needs are to be met by God. We have mistakenly given that "job" to someone else. There are three problems with that: 1) we did not notify him that he was fully responsible, 2) it is not his job, and, 3) he is not capable. My emotions are a full time job. He will need a break—one I cannot afford.

At any rate, we, including Bathsheba, need to remember the self-esteem is that element which needs upgrading. That upgrade comes from a better relationship with God. The self-esteem is a total package: longer skirts, better choices, and fewer life-altering consequences. Your dress communicates your reverence to God and your self-respect.

Your Attitude

"Talking like that, she can't be a Christian!" "If Christians behave that way, then I am better off not being one!" "Her mannerisms do not seem to be an example to others." Have these statements ever been made about you? Do you believe the promises of God? All the time? Is your faith ever shaken? How easily? How do you respond to adversity? Do you find yourself complaining? Do you question God

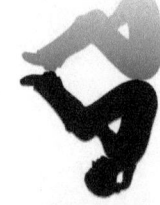

about the events in your life as if He has lost His directions? Do you pray daily? Do you meditate consistently on His word? Do you fast when you cannot function under His control? Do you fast when you cannot function under His control? Do you test Him with conditional statements you cannot possibly honor? Do you treat yourself and others poorly because your spirit is weak?

Our attitude determines how others see us. In this sight of us, they do not only see us but God in relation to us. The person making judgment on us and our relationship to God is using how they feel about what we as Christians should be doing. Is that fair? Maybe not. But what is fair is God's expectation of our attitude. Our attitude should exemplify the most intimate relationship and the ultimate in reverence to God. What does that mean? We are in charge of ourselves. We are responsible for our actions as a result of how we feel. Our attitude needs to show the best of God possible. How is that possible?

As I write this, many of us are faced with many issues and situations. The choice we make about how we respond is reflective on God, not just us. As you consider an issue or situation, ask yourself what is my attitude about that. Attitude is a noun defined according to dictionary.com as a manner or feeling with regard to a person or thing. The interesting point is that attitude is a noun, rather than a verb.

How can we show the best possible attitude? The best manner or feeling about each person or event or situation or thing.

Consider the following scenario: your boss is always "coaching" you. He never gives you any praise or accolades especially when you close the deal for the department which gathers recognition

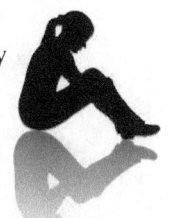

from the CEO of the company. Your boss holds you accountable at a higher level. You have to do everything. He is always asking of you. At some point, you wish not to see him coming, calling, emailing or any other communication. How can we not feel that way, although we may have be "justified?" Before we "dislike" him, can we ask him for the praise we desire to keep us motivated? Keep in mind that he asks you for several reason: 1) you are dependable, 2) you do great work, 3) he does not think you need praise, 4) you are being groomed for a promotion; and, 5) you have a great attitude!

Understanding others' motives requires a healthy attitude. That healthy attitude is developed from prayer and a growing relationship with God. The closer we grow to Him, the easier it is to have a pleasant attitude, how we may consider ourselves distant from the "less-than" attitude I recently described. Let's get a little deeper.

What do we do when someone who has harmed us, whether emotional, financial, political, comes into your presence? What do I do when someone who has continuously meant harm to me is in my presence? Does my attitude change? Do I change my demeanor? Am I openly hostile as a defense mechanism because of this person? Why do I allow this person to affect my attitude? Why am I indifferent when that person's name is mentioned? Why am I distant when that person speaks?

Why can't I love than with the love of Christ? Regardless of the actions of the other person? The flesh we inhabit is fragile and that "offense" is not easily forgiven and certainly not forgotten. We have a knack for remembering what someone did which offended us, the exact date, time, details, the weather and all other pertinent details. All of that

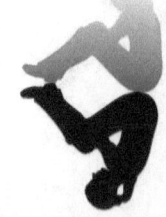

memory requires space. Your brain and memory is like a memory card yet worse. Your memory is limited and should only be used for important stuff. I have learned to release others from my accountability bondage. Likewise, I can release myself from that same bondage. I can use my memory for more scriptures, more writings, and more of whatever God wants.

Now, the greatest moment in this release is the realization that God has you. God is your protection and protector. He only gives you what you can bear and He uses these events and persons to draw you closer and add wisdom and perseverance to your life. There was a time in my life when I knew that He had me on solitary confinement. He had me completely alone. He had limited my access to everyone: family and socially, so that He could have my full attention. He also did that so He could protect me from the pain they could possibly bring and He needed my attention on Him for the next steps in my life.

With that in my mind, we have to forgive them and love them with the love of Christ. Likewise, out of reverence and obedience to Him, our attitude will be pleasant. A pleasant attitude communicates that God is in control. That pleasant attitude reminds that the distracter is not more important than God. They may be in "student" mode and you are being used at the example of how to handle adversity and unpleasant people.

Your positive attitude communicates to God that He is in control and that you trust His plan for your situation. Your positive attitude shares your faith despite the bleak outlook of your situation. Your attitude speaks loudly with the fear of God that you believe. Our best attitude draws others to God through us. Remember my reference

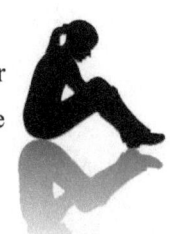

earlier to my verbal abuse of the sales associate. My attitude was not reverent toward God.

A good attitude does not harbor complaining, but optimism and good will toward all, especially those who seek your harm. A good attitude is a daily work—a journey, a process—not a destination. Your attitude is challenged daily, multiple times each day. The Bible says that it is easy to love who already loves you (1 John 4:19-21). Our charge is to love those who do not love us and those who are labeled as unlovable. A good attitude is a full-time participation-dependent job. It requires re-calibration daily, sometimes hourly, and sometimes, each minute. This means that it needs our focus and attention.

Your Praise and Worship

The last elements where fear of God should be completely evident are our praise and worship. First of all praise and worship is separate while equal. Each are equally important. They are different. They are often confused and mistakenly interchanged. Praise is defined as strong words of approval and worship of God. Even dictionary.com used them interchangeably. Worship is defined as a reverence for a god, adoring reference, and a formal expression of reverence. In this definition, praise is not mentioned. Praise is defined by Gage as the words and other verbal, or written expression to show and express adoration for God. Praise closes the gap between us and God, Jesus and the Holy Spirit because of sin.

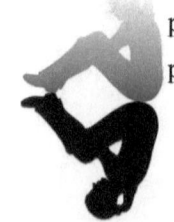

Praise is excellent at expressing the fear of God. Our words of praise to God through song, words of adoration, and confession give platform to our praise. We were made to praise God. He made us to adore Him for who He is and all that He has done. Often we discuss do not just praise Him for what He has done, but this not a material reference. In this context, 'done' is measured by creating the Earth, universe and the fullness thereof. Further, God gave us Jesus Christ then the Holy Spirit—He deserves our praise for Them being given to us. He created each of us—He deserves our praise. He has plans for us (Jeremiah 29:11)—He deserves our praise. He loves us unconditionally (John 3:16)—He deserves our praise. He forgives us for our transgressions, even when we do not forgive ourselves, especially when others do not forgive us (Nehemiah 9:17)—God deserves our praise. He provides for us (1 Timothy 6:17)—God deserves our praise. He gives us His peace (Philippians 4:7)—God deserves our praise. He lifts our spirits from the depths of what would be defined as depression but He never lets it get that bad (Psalm 40:1-3). God deserves our praise. He provides us with gifts such as preaching, teaching, singing, administration, and those gifts are to be used to further His kingdom (1 Corinthians 12:28)—His investment deserves our praise. There are thousands of reasons why He deserves our authentic, unadulterated and unconditional praise.

Yet out of disrespect or disobedience or discontent or total irreverence, we do not praise God. We praise Him with poor motives and in severe conditions. When I consider the lowest points of my life, I should praise Him for the glory He will receive when He restores me to where He wants and wills me to be.

We praise out of reverence! Let us discuss David once more. David is a great example of what happens when we praise God. David has plenty of opportunities to praise God and for various reasons to do

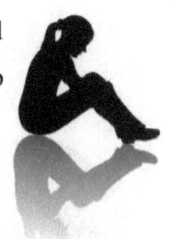

so. He shares so much of himself through the scriptures. David is the voice of most of the Psalms. The praises which we learn and claim as favorite scriptures are from David. Psalm 8:1: "O Lord, Our Lord, how excellent is thy name in all the Earth! Who hast set your glory about the heavens. (KJV)" This is one example of David's praise.

When we praise God, we share our reverence to Him and we express our gratitude to Him for His grace and mercy. Praise is a love note to God. When we praise God, others witness our reverence to God and our testimony may change the lives of others.

Worship is the action we do to adore God. These are acts of service to God, through sacrifice and the exercise of gifts given by God. Worship is designed to glorify God and complete His purpose.

Worship shares how we adore God. How do we worship? How does God know we adore Him? How do others know that I adore God? I worship through my service and my voice and behavior and my leadership. My worship exhibits my respect for God. Worship requires us to focus on God and only on God. I mentioned earlier that I had accidently put my ex-husband and children before God. To that end, God resolves that no one and nothing comes before God, Jesus nor the Holy Spirit.

Fear of His commands and His word are also applicable for reverence as well. God has to be respected, honored thus revered.

What we do not fear is other people and stuff. He does not give us a fearful spirit for other stuff. What we should not fear, we do. What we should fear, we do not. This would include the phobias. God

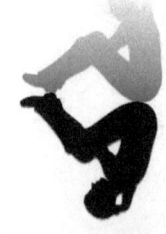

gives us several tools to overcome our fears. The first of which is when we live in fear of those who are supposed to love us. When we fear a person, that is the definition of an unhealthy relationship. This typically happens within spousal and familial relationships. Women who fear their husbands are often subjected to low self-esteem and poor handling, maybe even his physical and emotional abuse. There are other family members who are in fear of one or more family members because of the posture or occupation. Neither of these is by God's design. While this is to pray for that person to stop lording over you and prayerfully prepare for the releasing or reconciliation of that relationship.

Likewise, God has not designed others to fear you either. This fear is by choice or sub-consciously. Often I hear that I intimidate other(s). In this situation, I contend that intimidation is a choice. Likewise, I am responsible to insure that I do not take advantage of that person in their fears and otherwise weaknesses.

God does not regard fear well because our lives are exercises of faith because He said so. When we fear, we tell Him that we doubt Him, that we do not trust, that we do not believe, and we let fear reign in His place. God, Jesus and the Holy Spirit cannot co-exist in the same dwelling place as fear. To remove fear, prayer is required. We have to move decisively when we seek to abandon fear. This was different than the worldly view; which states that we are to make others fear us, or that there is nothing we can do about fear. Contrary to that myth, God, Jesus, and the Holy Spirit can relieve you of that fear. Jesus cast out demons a few times. There was a mutual fear: we are afraid of the demonic, and they are afraid of our judgment.

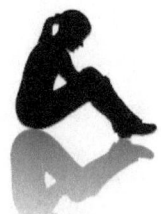

When you consider your fears, why do you fear that object or person? Why do you fear that? How long has that been your fear? What does it take to rid yourself of that fear? What does it take to transfer that inappropriate fear to a fear for God? When I consider the Spirit of power, the Spirit of love and the Spirit of self-discipline, I know that I must relinquish those fears. The Spirit of power will be tested by others and exercised by you. This requires focus—focus which does not work well with your focus on fear. The Spirit of love is always worth working on with others. I can increase those I love as well as the intensity with which I love. If I spent more time loving, I would not have much time for anything else, especially fear. The Spirit of self-discipline is all that we have to share which separates us from the animals and non-believers. Our self-discipline is critical for growth and certainly needed to overcome our fears. God will help us with our self-discipline if we lack the skills to employ it personally.

Pray to the Holy Spirit for help with your reverence of God, adjustments in what you fear, the spirit of power, of love and of self-discipline and anxiety await His deliverance.

Fear of God dictates a particular posture with Him. Our hearts must be humbled and pride-free and fertile for Him so He can do His best work within us for His glory.

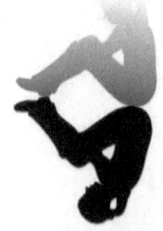

THE MIND FACTOR

⁷ And the peace of God, which transcends all understanding, will guard your hearts and your minds in Christ Jesus.

Philippians 4:7
New International Version (NIV)

² Do not conform any longer to the pattern of this world, but be transformed by the renewing of your mind. Then you will be able to test and approve what God's will is—His good, pleasing and perfect will.

Romans 12:2
New International Version (NIV)

The mind and brain are the processor to all information. The United Negro College Fund (UNCF) states that "a mind is a terrible thing to waste." This statement shares that minds or brains should be educated, cultivated, and expanded. The organization funds college education for the purpose of protecting those minds.

The protection that an education provides is quite different from what God desires for us. God wants our mind focused on Him, His work and His business. Your mind is a precision instrument. It is designed to make decisions, process and store information. This place cannot house junk well because it was not made for that.

God's plan is that we would keep our mind "stayed" on Jesus. There is an old spiritual that articulates this activity. God's definition of a mind which is yielded and submitted to Him is different from ours. God defines our minds focused on Him as not allowing distractions to distract our minds from Him. How do we do that? Great question. Two mechanisms He designed for this is: the word No and prayer.

God has plans for us. He reveals them to us on a need to know basis. And often we are notified of His plans right before it is time to start that assignment. God knows us and that means that He knows what our weaknesses are and what our apprehensions are. God knows what we are scared of and what will make us arrogant. Because of all that knowledge, God will share with us based on what we can handle and shields us from what we cannot. God shares with us when He knows that we cannot turn back from His plan.

Many of us cannot have choices or forks in the road. We will make the "flesh" choice each time. We need to master saying NO to the things that God does not want us involved in. Learning to say NO is hard because we will say NO to some exciting activities. We will be saying NO to things we previously said yes to. Previously this distracted us from God now we must say NO.

I cannot manage all of the areas that are presented to me where I should be saying NO but I say yes. Maybe you do not have that problem but if you do then you understand that NO is necessary. Saying yes detours us from the real plan and delays God's deserved glory.

Prayer is the tool we use to say NO more often than we would normally. Prayer is the only mechanism which helps to make NO happen and sustain that NO. Prayer is designed by God for part of that reason (refer to *The Prayer Factor* chapter).

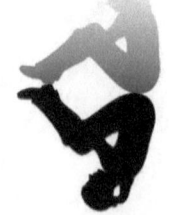

The composition of the mind is a collection of messages which are gathered over the course of our lives. The mind is interchangeable with the brain. For this study, I use mind because the brain technically is "blamed" with only the knowledge. The mind is the composed of the comprehensive experiences. I want to deliberately remind you that your knowledge is built both on knowledge which comes from book knowledge and knowledge developed by experience. These two details are developed into a "married" knowledge which is the content of your mind. Brain is the physiological element that monitors the body's behavior which transmits chemicals that dictates the actions we will take.

Our mind is pliable. Our minds can be changed. Our mind can be manipulated. Our minds can be bought with imagery. Our minds are the hubs of processing information. The mind decides whether we participate in events or sleep or learns. The mind determines who we greet or befriend. The mind decides who we like but the heart decides who we love. Sometimes those decisions are not aligned. Your mind makes decisions based on facts mixed with the results from an emotional activity. The mind remembers specific events which led to emotional pain or other such emotional mishaps. Because the mind remembers, the mind decides to avoid the future such events.

We have taken this path to illustrate the layers that compose the mind. These layers are protected by God so that your mind can remain focused on Him.

This is a relationship book. God spends lots of time and experiences convincing you that you deserve His love, that the disappointments are only healed by Him and He is the only one

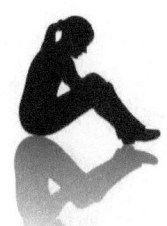

RESPONSIBLE for your complete protection and only His LOVE is conditional. The problem is He has to reprogram your mind in order for that to take place.

Now that we have established the basis of the ultimate relationship, we need to understand the scriptures.

The two questions I am asked often and for awhile asked myself: 1) What is God's peace like? and, 2) How can I know God's will for my life?

Peace is defined by Gage as the interruption-free sleep. It is the ability to remain calm when issues arise. Peace is also the understanding that God is in control and whatever happened is in His control. The situation does not require worry. Peace means that we do not immediately react or respond. Peace means that we seek God for guidance in these matters. Peace means that we wait on an answer from God without anxiety. Peace provides you the opportunity to relax in God's arms. This peace which transcends our understanding—I love the composition of this scripture—gives us power. His peace is not something we will understand immediately. God's goal is for us to have a peace which causes awe within ourselves. This peace is not something we can claim as what we did for ourselves which we would be quick to do. The word transcends gives the elevated impression that we may never understand the peace God provides. Dictionary.com defines transcends as 'to go beyond the ordinary limits of' and 'to surpass.' Consider this awesome peace that God provides is well-timed, well-placed, and extremely comforting—nothing that you would have done or thought for yourself. We cannot give ourselves the peace God gives us!

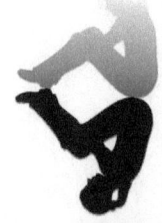

The cliché, I am going to give her a piece of my "mind," is often spoken in retaliation for a comment or activity which was not pleasing to the recipient. The problem is that the proverbial concept is that you are sharing your feelings. When you say this statement people may laugh because you have stated that you are going to give parts of your mind away. While you are not actually doing it, we need to consider giving others the PEACE of our minds.

Sharing God's peace from our hearts and minds is what we need to be equipped to do. This peace covers our hearts as well. God's peace provides protection. This protection guards against everything. Define everything, you may ask. Clearly you could think of some instances when you did not feel guarded, left unprotected. In these situations, you need to return to the Source. The Source—God—will place protection as we allow and only we can access.

God is motivated to protect your mind. God needs your mind to be focused on Him. The relevant activity we are to be engaged shares that our minds and our hearts are connected. Our minds and our hearts are both needed to be in sync with God so that we can serve Him the way He called us to do.

The "mind" makes decisions based on the expressions and experiences. The "mind" is a decisive place where many factors are considered before a final choice is made. The "mind" is a difficult entity to change and difficult to manage. When the "mind" had made its decision, the ability to influence change is limited. These limits are defined by persons whom the "mind" trusts, respects, and loves. The "mind" does not change for persons who do not possess a strong collection of all of those characteristics of influence.

The "mind" must trust the Source. The source has to be reliable and has a no or very small failure rate. The source has to have a track record of great results. At the point which the trust fails between the mind and the source, the source loses its influence. The "mind" will seek another source. The confusion for some is that the "mind" will choose an unknown source over a reliable source. The source appeals to logic of "mind." The logic has to match with current knowledge, and previous experience. At that juncture, the "mind" is establishing and reaffirming trust. As the trust grows, the greater the influence of the Source becomes.

The "mind" then has to respect the Source. Without the respect, the "mind" may listen but will not take action. This will confuse the source because the source was not notified of the lowering respect factor so the influence is lower than anticipated. Various events cause this reduction. The "mind" has to learn to articulate the respect level. The source was not aware that because the "mind" made "a note to self" and took the opaque road as a solution.

Lastly, love of the Source is the most detailed influence of your mind. Consider how we frame the word "love" and the definitions we attach to that noun, verb, and the adjective we indiscriminately use and often misappropriate. Love should not be so flexible as any part of speech. Likewise, love was firmly shared, shown, defined, and demonstrated.

We are so far away from the original definition that we doubt the path that could lead us toward the Source.

The "mind" changes only because of trust, respect and love. While this seems simple enough is a process from which to recover.

As we understand our "mind" and the state of our "minds," which includes an honest discussion with ourselves about the details which have contributed to the current situation, we are going to have to realize that our "minds" have to point to God. We have to start to eliminate the events and situations which have separated us from God. Our "minds" have to be made up to completely follow God so that we can reap the benefits of God's attention and plans.

Consider the "mind" in its decisive state paired with God's plan and provision. What would happen when you fix your "mind" on Christ? Totally fixated on Christ. At this very moment, your "mind" is divided between God and the world. God is in competition for your whole "mind." The problem is that He is not supposed to be in that type of competition. The fact though is that He is waiting on your submission and that submission is an invitation to God to the primary focus of our "minds." God does not need our consent or permission to occupy our whole "minds." God can do whatever He wants. He can summon me to Him whenever He wants for whatever He wants. The part we miss out on is that He ALLOWS us to be out of order until He tires of our self-inflicted foolishness which He has so often has to save us from. He is anxiously waiting for us to DECIDE to completely submit our MINDS to Christ. God made me and knows me so well. The fact is that He knows how strong I am and just how driven I am and just how much ambition I have and exactly what motivates me. God knows exactly what He will do to stop my mind from any further separation and lack of focus on Him.

The phrase your "mind is a steel trap" is normally used to reference the memory capabilities and the mental capacity. The phrase leads us to believe that what goes in does not come out. The very idea

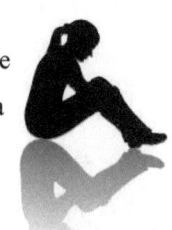

God is trying to avoid is the junk which occupies our "minds" to remain there. An enhanced relationship with God and growth moves that faulty information from the "steel trap" and reach for some better information.

God knows that the "mind" is the highest and most reliable source for a closer relationship with Him. God has to overcome so much garbage. The scripture affirms that we are already committed to Christ with our "minds" and hearts. The protection He provides is a measure for keeping us focused.

God is in competition for your "mind" with idols and sheer foolishness! How judgmental of the author to say that! Yes, because I have to start with me. What is on your "mind?" What occupies your "mind?" What is the content of your thoughts? Are you working on the "mind" of Christ? What does it take to eliminate the mental interruptions?

The images of your eyes become the images of your "mind" and those images become thoughts. What you see has the ability to consume your "mind." What are you listening to? What are you hearing? What is seeping into your "mind"—with or without your consent? The audible content plays over and over in your "mind" based on whatever triggers are in place to recall that audio. Consider music as an example. There are songs you learned years ago, some of them you learned as a child, and you can still sing almost every word. That song is learned. It is locked into your memory. It is in your "mind." So consider what you have taken in your "mind" and how that has molded your actions, attitudes, feelings, and thoughts.

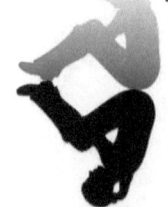

The "mind" drives all of these aspects. What we take in determines our character. So a man thinketh, so he is (Proverbs 23:7). This proverb clearly outlines that our thoughts determine who we are.

Part of your personal testimony includes things which are on your "mind," so I will share mine.

When I decided to lose weight because I weighed 204 pounds after the birth of my second child and my mate did not look at me anymore, I lost 50 pounds because I changed my "mind."

I was thirteen years old and I found myself underneath a pile of other teenagers. I had asthma at the time. At the bottom of the pile, I am having an asthma attack. After the end of the attack, I decided that I would never have another attack. I have not had another attack. I have not had a surgery. I am not on medication nor do I have a prescription for any. Because I made up my "mind."

At two years old, I was "allergic" to most of the items I loved or wanted, including a dog. On a regular visit to the pediatrician for more allergy shots, I informed the doctor that I was not taking any more shots. Because of my "mind."

I decided that I wanted to have more education. I researched, enrolled, and completed that degree. Three times. Because it was on my "mind."

When I understood and accepted God's calling on my life to minister as a preacher, I had to decide to understand that some family and friends would leave me because they did not agree with God that women could preach. Because God has my "mind."

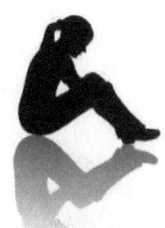

I decided to do those things as God blesses and provides. God created our "minds" to serve Him. I decided those things and was successful with God's blessings. Matthew 22:37 reads, "Jesus replied, "Love the Lord God with all of your heart and with all of your soul and with all of your mind.""

As it stands, I have demonstrated the "mind's" powers and abilities. You have similar stories. Likewise, when I serve God with this much decisiveness, God knows my love, respect and reverence for Him. As we consider the "mind" and the various paths it could take, we could have a poorly cultivated "mind" with dangerous intentions and actions, and not understand why this is not okay. God keeps us and our "minds" from faltering and failing, when He could let us continue down that path, however that path is not useful for Him.

The scripture states that we love God with all of our "minds." Our "minds" cannot be distracted because it is supposed to be ALL focused on God. How do we move those distractions, eliminate those unwholesome memories and thoughts, and eradicate those negative dialogues?

The answer is to renew your "mind"! Our second focus scripture is Romans 12:2. "Do not conform to the pattern of this world." Do not behave, think, act, feel, care, work, play, educate, worship or love like the rest of the world, which is brutally selfish, eccentrically self-centered, and bitterly driven toward the opposite of Christ. Avoid this at all cost! The fact is that the extreme image I present is highly avoidable. It is easy not to be completely unselfish. It is easy not to care about anyone but ourselves. But it is hard to avoid both of these.

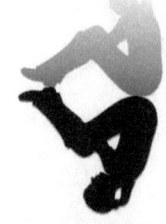

The reality is that the "middle of the road" is the real problem when keeping our "minds" renewed and focused on Christ. The extremes are never usually the problem because many of us are not brave enough to go to the extreme. It is that one or two degrees to the left or the right that usually causes the problem, where sin starts to enter and sometimes it stays.

In order to avoid the pattern of this world, we have to decide to do the opposite and differently. It is hard to be different. Many of us are afraid to be different. We seek the approval of others. The different ones do not concern themselves with the approval of others. I know that you may be saying that this is easier said than done. There are at least three occasions when you can recall when you knew definitely that God loves you. God's love is enough to make you reject the need for the approval of others. Consider carefully the times when God has loved you when others have rejected you. God deserves your full and undivided attention. That love includes the fact that depending on the approval of others has to be abandoned.

The next important part of renewing your "mind" is avoiding and removing the interferences which separate us from God. Avoiding sin. Avoiding distractions. Avoiding busyness. Avoiding avoidance. I am suggesting avoiding those images which have caused you to sin. I am suggesting the upgrade of your "mind" through what you take in.

What are you reading? Do you read? How much television do you watch? How much gossip do you share? Do you have all the education you need? Do you have gifts you are not using? How much time do you spend with God? Seeking God? What is on your "mind"? Are your thoughts related to God?

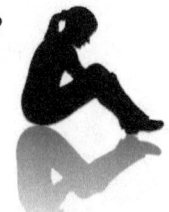

As we renew our "minds," we need to study and investigate what is important to God. We need to peel the layers of the onion of our lives to seek those places which we are serving God or not. Pray for the desire to do those things which are displeasing to God be weakened and eliminated. This will be a process, which starts with deciding to give up some things. Then the wise choice is asking for help. Lastly, participating in the process shares with God that you are serious about Him, His will, His Word, His work, and His plans for your life.

Renewing your "mind" also means that your hearing and vision will vastly improve. Does your "mind" make the God choice or otherwise? Does your "mind" respond in real time to the Voice of God, Jesus and the Holy Spirit? Renewing also means that you are not easily drawn away from God.

Renewing your "mind" means that you are better able to recognize the oncoming of sin. You are able to more easily avoid sin because you are more focused on God.

One of the patterns of this world is that God is used as a cosmic bellhop. We must avoid the temptation of this behavior as well as making deals with God. God desires a relationship with Him for who He is and not because of what He has done, can do, or will do. The renewal of the "mind" is one which studies and prays daily and is focused on God in such a manner where the evidence is visible outwardly.

Renewed "minds" show God on her face. When the smile and bounce is all about God and His awesomeness. And His goodness. And His mercy. And His grace. Renewed "minds" only speak wholesome

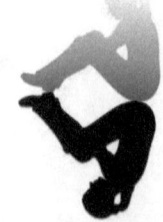

talk and wise words. This is an exercise of self-management and discipline. This is going to require your full engagement and focus.

A renewed "mind" is fresh. Your creativity is revived. You should be able to understand your spiritual gifts, where they are to be used and how to implement them at the church where you serve.

Your renewed "mind" is able to step away from the negative, even if it was self-inflicted. The negative discussions must stop right now. The lessons about this are numerous in the Bible. The woman with the issue of blood comes to "mind." I want to discuss the little engine, the blue one, the one from our childhood. I think I can. Never said I'm not so sure. Positivity is key to ALL success, inclusive, if not beginning with renewing your "mind." The woman pressed past the negative with her "mind" focused on Jesus—not anything or anyone else.

A renewed "mind" ignores any consequences related to focusing on God, or earnestly seeking Jesus or meeting the Holy Spirit. When I seek God, I am not concerned about what others are thinking about themselves or me. I cannot please God and man. I chose God because He ALWAYS chooses me.

A renewed "mind" shares openly about the desires and work of Christ. If we cannot share Christ with others, then there is shame or ignorance. When God is God, there is an urgency to share Him with others. There is a need to bless Him by telling others about Him—no matter if it does nothing.

A renewed "mind" and a changed thought pattern lead to being able to test God's will in your life.

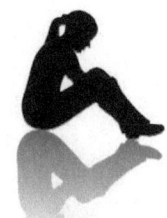

What is God's will for my life? This is a very popular question. Hearing from God and the vision God provides is the way we find out what God's will is for our lives. God is going to share His will and plans for us. We have to be focused to see it.

When I first committed to abstinence, I could discern better who was focused in my same manner. I was able to concentrate on my work assigned by God. Did it make my life perfect? Not in the manner you may be thinking but I was perfect to God. As a matter of fact, I divorced the man who presented himself as the person who understood my commitment. I learned to still TEST what is presented to me to insure if it is of God's will. Besides if it is for you, then you will receive it. You do not have to plan or plot, maneuver or manipulate.

Eugene Peterson, the author of the Message Bible, shares Romans 12:2 in this manner: "Don't be so adjusted to your culture that you fit into it without even thinking. Instead, fix your attention on God. You'll be changed from inside out. Readily recognize what He wants from you, and quickly respond to it. Unlike the culture around you, always dragging you down to its level of immaturity, God brings the best out of you, develops well-formed maturity in you."

A "mind" focused on God results in great progress in God's will.

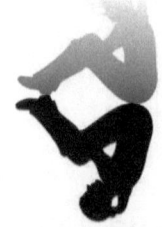

THE BODY FACTOR

[19] Do you not know that your body is a temple of the Holy Spirit, who is in you, whom you have received from God? You are not your own; [20] you were bought at a price. Therefore honor God with your body.

1 Corinthians 6:19-20
New International Version 1984 (NIV1984)

[16-20] There's more to sex than mere skin on skin. Sex is as much spiritual mystery as physical fact. As written in Scripture, "The two become one." Since we want to become spiritually one with the Master, we must not pursue the kind of sex that avoids commitment and intimacy, leaving us more lonely than ever—the kind of sex that can never "become one." There is a sense in which sexual sins are different from all others. In sexual sin we violate the sacredness of our own bodies, these bodies that were made for God-given and God-modeled love, for "becoming one" with another. Or didn't you realize that your body is a sacred place, the place of the Holy Spirit? Don't you see that you can't live however you please, squandering what God paid such a high price for? The physical part of you is not some piece of property belonging to the spiritual part of you. God owns the whole works. So let people see God in and through your body.

1 Corinthians 6:16-20
The Message (MSG)

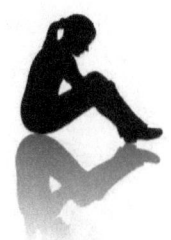

The body is a powerful organ. This instrument is used to serve God, work, love and serve others. This instrument was created by God from dust. He delivered us to this Earth to serve. No matter what the circumstances or the issues or the reason you were told you were born or how you arrived here, you were created to serve God with the body you have.

When we accepted Jesus as our Lord and Savior and invited the Holy Spirit into our hearts and to dwell within us, we committed to share our bodies with the Holy Spirit. Your body never belonged to you. That body is on loan.

The body we have is a testimony which people view as our connection to God. How we treat that body is a reflection of our relationship with God. We need to treat our body with the respect and dignity it deserves. In some areas, this may be harder than others.

Just as a caution, the following may seem judgmental and absolute, however it is the truth as presented by the Bible.

We are to guard our flesh from many things, which includes tattoos, piercings, weight, health, exercise, rest, water, appearance, abuse, and sex. Some of us consider our bodies are our own and we can do what we please to it but that is not the case.

Tattoos

Tattoos are not allowed. Whew! I spent a lot of time framing that sentence and it did not work any other way. They alter the body in ways not representative of God. "It's a cross." "It's just a butterfly!" You have altered the status of your body for recreational purposes. This

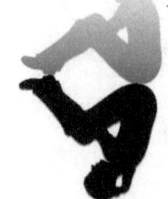

THE BODY FACTOR

is not of God's will. I know that if you have tattoos or your children do, this is hard to read or see.

I have taught my children not to get tattoos for two reasons: (1) because it displeases God, and, (2) skin graphing is expensive. If there is the potential that you are not going to always feel the same way about that person or place or thing, then we should avoid that moment. The regret and remorse is immeasurable. The constant explanations about why did you get that tattoo and what does that mean. The actual and potential discrimination from employers and mates is already experienced by many. At some point, you will be a grandmother and you may want to teach otherwise, however the weight of your message is diminished because young people do not follow the "use my experience to avoid repeating my mistakes." They view the fact that you did "it" and survived to share it then it is not a big deal to them that you would rather they make a different choice.

Body Piercing

Body piercings follow this same activity. So should I have my ears pierced—if only once? No. That includes the author. It is an accepted practice when done in moderation however it still should not be done. We judge others who have move piercings or in unacceptable places or too numerous. Yes, the holes may close but there still may be a mark.

Weight, Health, & Exercise

Weight is a battle as big as the potential of World War 3. Weight loss pills and equipment and diets and programs are a billion dollar business. Your weight is not designed to be an obsession. Your

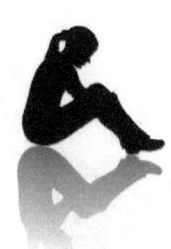

weight is a measure of health and reflects your self-image. There is a formula online suggesting what your ideal weight should be. This is a guide. Seek your doctor about what your ideal weight is. Then ask for a REALISTIC plan to reach that goal and how to maintain that goal.

Most of America is overweight. Childhood obesity is out of control and rising. Weight is driven by two factors: eating and exercise. Eating too much and exercising too little. Let me explain that eating too much is so common that we do not recognize when we do so. It is easy to rationalize that you did not eat too much.

Work to eat only half of the food at the restaurant. Put the other half in a carryout container. Eat that half when you are hungry again. We are concerned about wasting food. I am concerned about "waisting" food. This means that I would rather discard the food than let it settle on my waist. A friend said to me that I don't want the food to go to waste. My response was that I do not want it to go to my waist. When we can get past the distinction then weight loss and management will be easier. The best approach is to change your mind about food and eating.

For many of us, we eat based on a need for comfort. This is emotional eating. We eat when we are not hungry. We eat because we are happy, sad, angry, frustrated, and any other emotion we can use as an excuse to eat. We eat for every holiday, victory and special occasion. There are people you know who plan to overeat based on what is being cooked and who is cooking.

Eating is designed to nourish you and sustain you. When was the last time you were actually hungry? How long were you hungry? My point is that we eat to cope with _____. You complete that

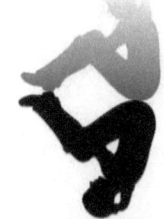

sentence with whatever it is you eat because. The goal is to move away from eating to coping to addressing the issue(s) with and through God.

Weight is inhibitive on your self-esteem as well as impacts your activity. Weight is serious because it impacts other factors of your life. Consider the option of losing a few pounds. Again access the power of your mind to lose the necessary pounds to progress to a necessary place.

Weight leads us to health issues. Your health is important. Your weight can negatively affect your health. You get one body! You cannot afford to treat it poorly! You only get one! You should do well to take care of the ONE you were gifted with! Your weight can drive your body parts to overwork and that overworking can wear it out.

There are people who are diagnosed with diabetes, heart disease, high blood pressure, and kidney failure. Some are diagnosed with cancer in its various formats. Any of these ailments could be changed by a gain of ten pounds. These additional ten pounds can and does make the heart work harder. Your health is a TOP priority. You cannot change the course of some illnesses. You can only manage it. There are some issues like cholesterol and high blood pressure which can be aided by diet and exercise, sometimes coupled with medication.

This body is the only one you get. Your health is critical to your relationship with God. Healing is a waiting moment which is truly a test of what God does in your life. There are things which we do sometimes which cause some of our problems: overeating, no water, smoking, no exercise to name a few. Then there are health issues which occur but we do not have control over it and did not do anything which led to that issue. There are illnesses which we are spared from and there is healing we benefit from. In those situations we need to consider what God has planned for you because He healed you **with** a testimony. When God gives you favor on your health, He has designed that healing to share with others through you. Your life is not to be lived casually as a child of God. There is an extra portion of grace when you have been kept here while you live with the "death sentence" you have been given by doctors and God proved them wrong.

Keep focus on your health because your body belongs to God. It was made to serve, house, and testify for God.

Your weight matters to God because it impacts how you feel about yourself. Your weight matters to God because it affects your attitude and openness toward others. God cares about your weight because it changes the way He made you.

Your weight, when not in control, invites others to criticize you and discriminate against you. Your weight could be hindering your witness. When I birthed my second child, I weighed 204 pounds. I was 60 pounds overweight. I could not wear much in my closet. I could not see the problem. Then I saw a picture of the back of my thighs and I saw a picture before my first child. Those pictures represented two different women! I woke up one morning and decided that the "fat" woman had to leave. She was overtaking me. She was not loving or lovable. She hated clothes because her pretty ones did not fit anymore. I called a weight program at the hospital and lost 51 pounds in four months. I was alive again. I could seek God, share Him with others and I was able to return to my calling, which I had abandoned because I could not face "her."

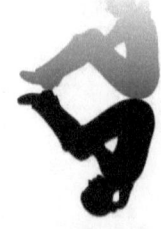

Lose the weight. Get some help. Pray for the motivation to take the necessary steps. I am praying for us. Weight loss is hard at best! God is required—the total sufficiency of His grace. Also, you need a REASON for this change, this lifestyle change.

I know my health history for my family for the most part. Because of that I do not eat pork. Yes, I did. I asked for God's help and He delivered me. So no, I do not have ribs at barbeques, bacon at breakfast nor ham at holidays. I do not miss or even crave it. Thank You, God!

This is about commitment and relationship. It is about decisions and sacrifice. It is about our best for God. We all know that weight breeds discrimination. Ask yourself what your weight is keeping you from achieving and being invited to or doing. Be honest. PRAY. Take action. Believe.

Exercise releases endorphins. Endorphins are the source of happiness. Endorphins are blamed for enhanced appetites and attitudes.

Exercise helps the weight loss, body maintenance and health. Research the appropriate regimen for you. Research the target heart rate you need to reach the optimum weight loss through the calories burned during each workout period. The normal is about 45 minutes to an hour of cardiovascular activity. This is optimum time so that the target heart rate can be reached so that weight loss can be achieved. More importantly your consistency is required. Four to five days each week until you reach your goal then you may reduce to three to four days as maintenance.

Get an accountability partner. This is someone who can help you when you are discouraged and need a lift. This person keeps you from cheating and quitting. Set goals and share them with those you can count on for REAL support. If you do not have anyone, send them to me at onediagage@onediagage.com. Decide. Do it. Lose weight. Triumph over your pain. Resume a relationship with God empty of shame!

Sleep and Rest

Sleep! Relax! Rest! This is not time for your start laughing. Yes! I mean you! I mean for you to rest! Eight hours each night! You are thinking impossible! I am not. Weight loss occurs during sleep. The body recovers during sleep. Sleep also helps your attitude and disposition. Rest revives and rejuvenates you. We are caught up in the busy and the hurry and the speed and the instant. Sleep requires time that you need to reallocate back to sleep rather than _____. Whether it is television, that PHONE, that INTERNET, that PHONE, put it down and SLEEP!!!

I have several friends who program their phones to automatically turn off at midnight and cut on in the morning. They have done that so that they are not disturbed in their SLEEP!!

Take a relaxing, warm bath! Drink some SLEEP tea! Go to SLEEP!!! Your rest determines your productivity. You cannot be productive without rest. The success you desire is related to rest.

I have fallen asleep in meetings, in church, and sometimes driving because I REFUSED my body some much needed rest. There are two issues which make me unbearable and irritable: SLEEP and

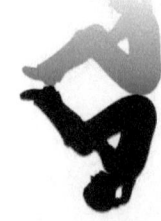

HUNGER. You are probably in that same category. You probably have these same characteristics. At any rate, SLEEP is critical. The sleep offers an opportunity to lose weight as well. Sleep offers so much more than what it appears to do. Go to SLEEP!

For successful sleep, I have some suggestions: sheets with 350 or higher thread count, bathe in a soothing fragrance, comfortable, soft pajamas, no television or laptop in the bedroom or in the bed.

The sheets are for a comfortable, cool sleep. The higher thread count makes the sheet smoother. There are fragrances with contain eucalyptus and chamomile. These ingredients are known for their calming effect. "Pajamas" have varied definitions. Comfort is the key. Figure it out. Lastly, the suggestion of no television in the bedroom or laptop in the bed is a rule I break regularly. Research shows that your brain needs to have time to stop moving as fast as your daytime pace. I am GUILTY of this so I have justification: I sleep well. I should follow my own advice better, and I am working on doing better. I fall asleep with the television on. I have moved my laptop to another room.

Practice sleeping better with better conditions. Lastly, studies show that you should replace your mattress every eight years. Good luck on sleep!

Water

This is the least favorite subject of most people: WATER! Many people hate water because of the lack of taste. Most of us prefer soda, tea, lemonade, and other drinks. Consider the calories, caffeine and other additives.

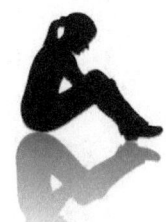

The "water rule" is half of your body weight in ounces. For example, if you weigh 200 pounds, then you should drink 100 ounces of water. DAILY. Catch your breath! Now the average water bottle contains sixteen ounces of water so that means that six to seven bottles of water. I prefer Ozarka. You can try all of the ones on the market or put lemon or lime in your tap water.

Consider the calories you eliminate when you eliminate some of these other sugar-based drinks by replacing them with water. Consider if you drink six to seven sodas each day. The twelve ounce can is 150 calories for Sprite. Six of those equal 900 calories. Your daily intake of calories for everything you consume is 1500. You just drank two-thirds of your calories. This could result in major weight loss if you replaced those sodas with water.

Water helps your overall health. A large, very large portion, of your body is composed of water. Somewhere near 90% of your body is water. Your whole body is dependent on water. Your body's thirst cannot be met with soda, liquor or any other liquid, other than water.

Dehydration can be deadly. Water is necessary. DAILY. I was pregnant with my second child and I was unaware that I was not drinking enough water. My doctor told me that if I did not get it together, that he would park me in the hospital. Water is critical to your life.

A last note: you were born in a water-based solution to be kept alive while in your mother's womb. Water is a solution to many issues. Please start a little at a time if you cannot eliminate sodas totally. At least match: for each soda, etc, then take a water along with it.

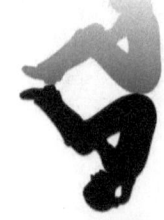

THE BODY FACTOR

DRINK WATER!!!

Clothing

Clothing is for the covering for the body. It is now the center of fashion. Fashion is a multi-billion dollar industry each year. We are addicted to clothing, fashion news, and "what am I going to wear?"

Why is this factor or detail important? I am glad you asked. Clothing is on your body and your body is the subject. Presenting your body to the public is something that you should take care of carefully. Your clothing speaks for you. Your attire speaks before you ever open your mouth. What does your attire really say? Does it say sleek, and sophisticated or athletic and grungy? Now let us not be misled. I am not judging either. I am offering however we pick how the world views us, judges us and treats us. Yes, we do! You see you make the choice each time you select clothing. You decide by your choices what people have the opportunity to say or think or feel or judge you by the outfits you wear.

There is a small faction of our society which thinks that you should be able to wear whatever you would like and there should be no consequences. Well please be assured those who think this is okay, then I want to authentically share that people judge you by your complete appearance.

Let's examine a hypothetical scenario: Imagine me wearing pajamas or shorts or sweats on the cover of this book or my website. What would you think? Would you respect me? Would you question the validity or integrity or authenticity of my message? Would you

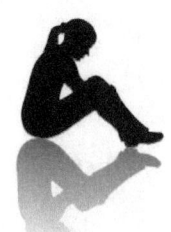

question if my information is valuable or reputable? Would you consider my education against my attire and ignore my attire?

The fact is that most of us cannot answer these questions. We do not want to answer them or think that we are that person who judges others based on what they wear. We are conditioned for this. Again we mentioned that billions are spent on clothing each year.

I select a professional image. One where people seek me because of the clothes I wear. Once they come to me, I can do God's work. It does not matter that people are drawn to me because of my cute outfit. When people judge you, you need to be author of their script. I decide what you say about me! Not you! I do not give you an ammunition that I do not want you to use.

I do not wear clothes that are too tight, too revealing, or too short. I do not wear clothes which cannot be worn everywhere. I do not leave home in hair rollers or anything which offers me an opportunity to WISH I had done differently. This is important because you express how you feel in your attire. When you are feeling low or down, that is when you want to dress up and be nicer than usual. You do not need any extra "bad" attention. When you feel "like death warmed up," you cannot feel better if someone confirms that you look "like death warmed up." When you do not feel your 100%, either stay at home or dress better so that someone does not feel licensed to confirm your feelings. When you look good, you will be complimented and your "blue-ness" will be overlooked. "Is that like faking it?" I am glad you asked. No, it is not. It is not being transparent in front of those who are not equipped to edify or uplift you in your time of need.

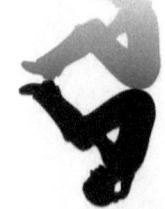

Now as for too tight. If your clothes are too tight, there are two reasons: you bought them too tight or you have gained weight so now they are too tight. If we have gained weight, then we need to stop wearing those garments until we lose that weight. If you bought it tight on purpose, what message are you sending? As a Christian woman, we have to guard the image of our body to others.

We want to be attractive but not in a lustful manner. I like attention but I do not want to dress in a manner that blatantly causes a man to sin in his thoughts.

Regarding the too revealing clothing, that philosophy is aligned with the too tight. Why am I calling that much attention to myself? I exercise discretion. I consider my body a gift and everyone cannot have access. When we consider our bodies as a treasure rather than a trading mechanism, then we feel better about ourselves. Always ask what does this outfit say about me? Would I be uncomfortable if someone I truly respected saw me wearing this outfit? If I am uncomfortable in this, then this is not the right outfit.

The too short outfit again is a matter of discretion. Give yourself permission not to subscribe to the hype to show it all.

A few last words about clothing: (1) define sexy; (2) define sexy regardless of the type of clothing; (3) is your attitude sexy? (4) when you are dressing for someone else, you will be subject to their subjectivity. That is too much dependence on someone else. (5) People respond to you based on your attitude about you; and, (6) most men I have spoken to about this matter suggest that we leave something to the imagination.

Most men do not want to see all of your assets. Keep something to yourself. For yourself. Your respect. Your self-worth. Your worth. All of that is worth wearing appropriately sized clothing. Discretion is our best presentation. We are charged to take care in our presentation of ourselves. Our bodies are important instruments for God. We need to understand the purpose of our bodies so that we can serve God appropriately! Clothing is key to that service.

Physical Abuse

This is a special topic for me. Domestic violence is a horrible situation for anyone. The state of mind of the two people involved is not normal. He is trying to exercise abnormal control. She is trying to be less of herself so that he can be comfortable in some poor excuse of himself. As a child, I witnessed my father hurt my mother. I promised bodily harm to a man so that he understood the consequence to such activity. This is not easy to do because we want to hold onto our man. I understand it. I really do. What I can do and what other women can do about this matter is different.

Your body belongs to God. It does not belong to him. If this is your situation, your first step is to pray in a confessional manner to God, sharing with Him your guilt that you feel that this is your fault. Research shows that victims feel that she is the reason for her abuse. This is not true. You are not responsible for his issues. He has ISSUES for which you are NOT responsible.

The second act is to forgive yourself. Then forgive him.

The third act is to WALK AWAY.

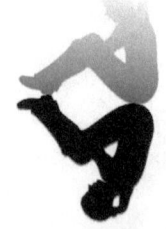

The fourth step is to receive God's LOVE: His pure, unconditional, true love. Better love than ever humanly imagined or conceivable. This is the love which makes your tragedy seem so different and the love is so profound that once you have immersed yourself in His love you may find yourself wondering how this ever happened to you.

The last step is to share your experience with others. When you are able to sharing your testimony with others, God is glorified! The devil is defeated when we share your testimonies and triumphs. No, it is not going to be easy, however we are to lift one another up and edify one and spur one another on in love. The women who will help are already waiting to hear from you.

Your body is designed to serve God. Make sure that happens properly.

Sex

This is a dangerous topic. This is an off-limit topic at best but we are going to discuss it. It will convict while it may not convince.

Sex is ordained for marriage. Sex is only for the married people to each other. Stop practicing. I know it is hard because it is your "go-to." The activity that you go-to when your day goes poorly or for whatever reason. There was an episode of Grey's Anatomy where Meredith told Lexie that her heart was in her vagina.

I have shared that on many occasions that our self-esteem is linked to whether or not he sleeps with you. You have graded your personal worth and value based on whether he is sleeping with you and hopefully not others simultaneously.

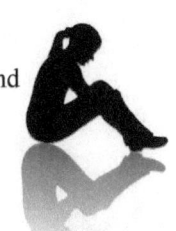

Sex has been proven to cause lack of judgment, especially in unhealthy relationships. The sex is good enough to keep you there. Seems strange to see that in writing but if you are honest there are some relationships which would not be a relationship if sex were not happening.

The statement about your heart being in your vagina means that you equate the sex you have to your emotional fulfillment. The first problem with that process is that you are a woman. He is not. You are driven by frilly and fru-fru. Yes, I am a woman. Yes, I am being transparent. He is not considering what your thought process was to arrive at "Yes, I will share my body with you." You said yes. He was excited. You had made that decision thinking that you were exclusive. He did not necessarily agree to that. To him, sex was an act. To you, it was affirmation.

We as women, would do well to consider that we make two decisions too quickly: (1) to whom to be committed; and, (2) with whom we sleep. For us, these decisions are one in the same. We have great intentions but we make some horrible decisions. With the benefit of hindsight, we see the error of our ways, however, we continue to make some of the same poor choices.

The point I am making is let us correct the problem. Stop seeking affirmation from a man. Stop using sex to lure, entertain, bargain or reconcile with any man. The problem is everybody is using sex to get at your man. Most men are propositioned all the time, often enough to get his attention, and other times he has no clue. At any rate, this is not a lasting method and in the long-term ineffective. And the short term.

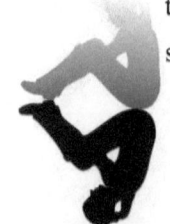

So that we do not get off track, this is a reminder that this is not a how to keep your man message, but rather how to reconnect with the most important MAN: God, Jesus and the Holy Spirit.

Sex is sin when you are not married. Sin separates us from God.

Protect your body even from yourself.

I have taught and advocated for abstinence for years. There were particular times when I was not. I want to talk about when I was though.

The first time I was able to say no was powerful. I told a guy I was truly interested in no. There was never a relationship after that. That kept happening too. I would meet a man. We start to get to know each other. Sex would come up. I would say no. He would be gone shortly, if not immediately. This happened repeatedly. Now realize that I was able to think and see clearly that each of them was not for me. Because we were not having sex, it was easier to walk away and know why I was walking away.

I realized that the sex had interrupted my self-esteem and self-image. I had to realize that it was important that I know my value and my worth. I had to know how important my relationship with Christ was—is. I had to reconcile that my heart and my vagina were always going to be connected. If I did not want to be hurt then I should stop giving away the treasures. I was giving away the body that God gifted to me. I was causing it pain and stress and drama. None of which it deserves or needs or can sustain.

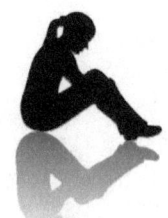

It is hard when you like sex or you are trying to like him or convince him to like you. Ask yourself would you marry him. If the answer is no, then why should sex be part of the agenda.

If you are going to sin, which I am not suggesting or advocating, then make it count, make it count with the man of your dreams. All sin is weighted the same so make it count. I say that because the opposite is what is really happening.

You give yourself away to the worst man and you are deeply angered by your behavior then you feel worse about yourself than before.

Keep in mind that I am suggesting that you reach for the stars: a man who respects you, knows your worth, understands your value and keeps you safe, even from himself. If he does not meet your criteria, you have sinned in VAIN.

We have each sought approval in the arms of a man. We have each thought if we have sex, he will like me more. If we have sex, I will have him and he will be committed to me. Has any of that ever been true? Has any of that profited you?

Someone once told me you can get more from the "promise of sex." Initially, I thought that type of misleading behavior could be dangerous. What that highlights is that when you have sex, you give away control to him. He knows and you do too. He knows you are emotional about the topic. He knows that he can use and manipulate that as a tool for what he wants.

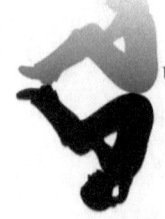

At any rate, the key is that your body is God's property, to be used for Him, by Him. We interrupt His work when we do the opposite.

How Do I Honor God With My Body

How can I do this?

On a regular basis?

Where others are motivated to do the same?

You get one body. It may serve you best to keep it functioning properly.

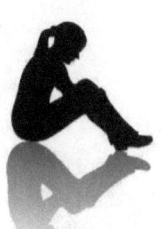

YIELDED AND SUBMITTED

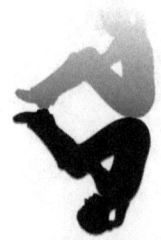

THE LIFESTYLE FACTOR

²²But the fruit of the Spirit is love, joy, peace, forbearance, kindness, goodness, faithfulness, ²³gentleness, and self-control. Against such things there is no law.

Galatians 5:22-23
New International Version (NIV)

"I live a life such that God is glorified in everything I do." She spoke this with confidence and conviction and cause. This is a challenge for many of us. Our lifestyle choices create problems and distance with us and God. Our lifestyle is a choice we make. God offers us His guidelines coupled with "the appearance of free will."

Gage defines lifestyle as simply how you live. The lifestyle we chose to live is a legacy we leave. The choices we make last awhile—and the poor ones last longer. With the invention of the internet and search engines, your deeds, hence your lifestyle, will last longer than you plan. Choose carefully so that a great lifestyle may result.

What are the rules of your life? What are the boundaries of your life? What are the standards in your life? What are the foundation pieces of your life? Who knows that those standards exist in your life?

First of all, God gave you a standard. Sometimes we set that standard aside. Let us understand that the standards are for God's usefulness. So let us define standard. Gage defines standards as what she will do and what she absolutely won't do. NO DRUGS. NO PORK. NO SMOKING. NO LAZINESS. NO DRAMA. Education is quite important as well. The bottom line is people decide who you are based on the standards you share.

When I was in college, my roommates knew that I would not drink with them. They knew not to ask about drugs. When they went to parties, they knew not to invite me to some parties and then those they did invite, there would be some modifications made. There was one toga party where I did not know exactly what that meant but what I did understand that the intent was to be nude underneath. I chose to wear clothes. They knew that was what I would do. They were also not surprised that I left earlier than they did. They knew that was my lifestyle.

Your lifestyle is defined by who you are and what you do and what you say.

Biblically, lifestyle is defined as the fruit of the Spirit. The fruit is what the Spirit is what the Spirit produces out of us. The fruit are nine elements functioning as one inside each of us. They are peace, joy, love, long-suffering, gentleness, self-control, faithfulness, goodness, and kindness. All of the details of the fruit have to be present as they are treated as a unit rather than separate pieces. We will discuss them separately though.

Love

Love is mentioned first. Love . . . what a word, what an example. Love is a verb. Love is defined as an action, an activity. If you love someone, there should be some evidence. There should be a result of your love on others. There should be some residue when you have loved someone. Love is a mystery to most of us. We cannot love

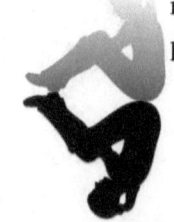

authentically because we have never been loved authentically. Authentic love is condition-free. Most of us have never experienced unconditional love. So then there is Jesus, The DEFINITION of Love. The ultimate definition of unconditional love. His actions from birth to death and every breath in between define love for us. From prayer to feet washing to healing to teaching, Jesus demonstrates love in its complete format. Jesus shares with us a love God designed.

How can we be that definition (or least close)? It starts with a decision. A decision to love. I have to decide to be loving to myself, God and others. How do we arrive at that decision? "Love is worth the effort." That is what I say to myself over and over. God is worth my love. I am worth love. Others are worth love.

So we have decided to love and we have determined that we are worth it, now we have to do two things: forgive and release. Love requires forgiveness. I am always challenged with forgiveness, of myself and others. In order for authentic love to exist, forgiveness has to happen. Ask God to help you to forgive. You may not be strong enough to do so alone. Be willing to forgive. Know that it is necessary. Now assuring that we can work through that, let's move on to love.

Love is verb and a noun. It is an action and an attitude. Love is an exercise of faith. You have to have faith what you will be loved in return or at least you will not get hurt in the process. Your faith and trust rests with God and not the person you are to love. Understanding that He is your comforter even if you are hurt.

Love is a result of deposits from the Spirit. Love exists within you because the Spirit deposited it there. The Spirit made that deposit so that you could love God, yourself and others.

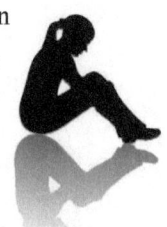

YIELDED AND SUBMITTED

Love is not a limited resource. It is quite limitless. We just have to understand our capacity. We are to love as a command from God. Matthew 22:37, 39 and John 13:35. Clearly He has supplied us with the love we need so that we can LOVE the persons who cross our paths. There are people, thousands of them, who will come in your path. You are designed and equipped to love them but you are too broken to do so. The forgiveness and consequently, the healing are necessary for the purpose of the love, and the usefulness for others. Our charge as Christians is to love and edify each other.

How do people know that you are love? How do you know that they can approach you for the love they need? How do you know who to love? What does love look like? Do you look like love? Does your face, tone, voice, words and body language speak love?

As an emotional human being, I consider myself gifted that I love with heavy emotion. The love I have and express to others is powerful and overwhelming. There is no question that I have the demeanor to love. There are times that my personality and presence intimidates and overwhelms others. So how do I manage this? It is difficult at best however, here are some pointers.

Consider your thought when you are approached or approaching others. What is on your mind? This may be written all over your face. When you have that pensive, thoughtful look on your face, you should consider smiling as the person who needs your specific version of love. The love that others need is the residual of the compassion of your story. They need the remnants of your love from tests of your life. They need the relief of love through the knowledge that your storms ended and a great outcome resulted.

If you notice that I used the words residue and remnants, so that means that people really do not need all that you have. They just need a little of your never-ending, God-given love. God renews your love and others are the beneficiary. As you share your love, you expand your witness. As you expand your witness, your heart grows. As your heart grows, you better understand the fullness of God. Your love shares a portion of God with others.

Our charge is to look like love, feel like loving others, especially when you do not want to, and share love without reservation because you are not on a love budget. God gave it to you in a limitless supply so that you can give it away.

When you love others, you show them Jesus. "It is the God in me" are lyrics made popular by a 2011 hit which is exactly what others are thinking. Both Christians and non-believers and non-Christians judge us for our love factor. "If that is how a Christian is then I do not need to be one" versus "I was loved by total strangers."

Your love can change a life.

Are you available?

Joy

Joy is one of the shortest and most peculiar words. It is so because the meaning is so big. Joy is the emotion of great delights or happiness caused by something exceptionally good or satisfying as defined by dictionary.com. In this definition, joy, delight, and happiness are used interchangeably. Joy is not defined that way in the Bible. Joy given by the Holy Spirit is not based or anchored in emotions. Joy is the result of a submission to the Holy Spirit. A

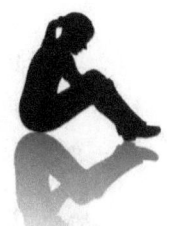

submission into the Holy Spirit. Once you realize that joy is a permanent expression rather than a fleeting emotion, it is easier to comprehend.

Gage's definition based on Biblical context is deeply anchored expression within you of an authentic encounter with the Holy Spirit which permeates through your words, deeds, body language and countenance. If joy is present and exists within you, there will be evidence.

As we measure whether someone or you have joy or are joyous, we consider a person's countenance, behavior, and reactions. There are several questions which are important. Is there an obvious edginess to the person's voice and facial expression? Is smiling a production? Are people always asking if you are okay? Do you need to have a moment to gather yourself? What is the predominant expression on your face? Does the smile you display emit warmth? Are people drawn to your attitude? Do people remark about your glow? Are your words seasoned and classy? Do people ask about your energy Source? Are you always tired? Do you allow things to bother you for a long time?

The answers are important to measuring your joy and how to achieve joy. I mentioned earlier an authentic immersion in the Holy Spirit, total submission with the Holy Spirit is how joy is attained. The same method is used to maintain.

Joy is evident on your face, in your words, in your heart, in your behavior, and in your mind. Your mind produces all of those things. So if you have joy in and on your mind, then that joy will have joy in all of your days.

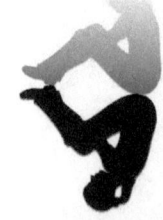

Once I understood joy, I was able to identify that I am a joyful person and can be looked to share that joy with others. Joy is an investment.

Peace

Peace. Rest for your soul. Relief from weariness. God's peace which transcends our total understanding (Philippians 4:7). Peace is a verb and a noun. Peace is desired. Being peaceable requires a peaceful disposition. Peace is an irreplaceable experience. Peace during your storms. Peace during your victories. Peace is the calm which reigns over your situation—no matter how seemingly horrible.

Peace is the relief we all desire when we do not see an end in sight. Peace is the rest for you to sleep through the night. Peace is the residue after the start of the storm when you wipe your brow and say, "Whew." Peace is the smile on your face while the storm is still brewing and the winds are 200 per hour. Peace that is not supposed to happen because the measure of the storm is so heavy that your spirit is supposed to be BROKEN.

'And the peace of God' . . . God is the author and originator of peace. His peace is what brings comfort and clarity, which transcends all understanding . . . This answers the questions 'how can you be this calm' and 'how does she do it with all that she has going on' and 'what are you going to do now that you are not working' and 'when are you going to find a job.' The peace that keeps you calm when you should be hysterical. The peace that allows you to remain sane and continue smiling when you should be shedding tears that would resemble hurricane-style rain.

'Will guard your hearts and your minds in Christ Jesus' . . . God is our protection from all stuff and storms, whether from enemy or self-imposed. The protection which God provides is like Fort Knox: secure, solid protection, which requires a mastermind to even consider trying to breach the package. God is protecting the critical areas: our emotional decision maker and our objective decision maker. God protects those two objects because that is how we are attacked, attached, and persuaded. This protection is to preserve us for Him. This is going to be mutually beneficial but He needs us whole and healing through our brokenness and hurt.

Keeping our minds and hearts in Christ Jesus is insuring that we don't wander away from Jesus Christ and remember to trust Him MOST during trouble. God knows exactly how much protection we need as well.

Being of peace and peaceful requires the guarding of God. Only God can bring forth the attitude and behavior which we label as peace. Peaceful is being calm during situations which are designed to stress and to hurt and to pain, to break and bruise and to empty.

Forbearance

Forbearance or long-suffering is the ability to withstand injury, trouble, provocation and insults with patience and perseverance.

It means to never quit during your hard times. My theme is "there ain't no quit me." Translation I won't quit. I am not made to quit. I am made to stand and I am made to fight. If you quit, God loses. God cannot get the same glory if you quit.

We have to stay in the fight.

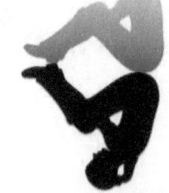

THE LIFESTYLE FACTOR

The best illustration of how forbearance or long-suffering works is a piano or violin. These are stringed instruments. The strings are responsible for the sound, the music which the instrument emits is made because the strings are pulled tight, placed with tension, positioned and equipped for tension. Let's make this really clear: without the tension, stress and tightness of the string, there would be no music! Without some stress, you would not make a joyful noise out to the Lord nor would you seek to serve Him any better.

I have to experience some things. I have to suffer through some things so that I can have the testimony to help others through their issues.

Long suffering proves to you what God knows you can withstand. Long suffering defines the authenticity of our lives. If we have not ever survived anything, then we hinder the extent of our praise and worship.

Forbearance is a tool God uses through us to attract others to us so that our lives will draw them to Jesus. He uses our "stuff" so that He can grow others.

Forbearance is not pleasant. It is the requirement of pain. But it is necessary.

Further, consider how proud you will be when you have met the expectations of God through what He believes you can do, far above what you ever consider yourself capable of and worthy of.

Forbearance is a portion of the fruit from the Spirit.

Kindness

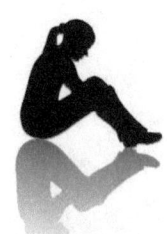

Kindness is an interesting fruit. Many of us are not kind to others because we do not know them. When we are not kind to others just because we do not know them, we are foolish. I notice in the work place that the more bad information we have, we have a pseudo-compassion because of someone else's misfortune.

Be kind because in this life we each deserve the other's kindness. Life is hard enough without someone being MEAN to you because they don't know you. Conversely, you are kind to people you do not like because of what you hope they will do for you or what they have done or what they have "promised" to do or what they are capable of doing.

Jesus is expecting that we are kind to others regardless of the details or facts or your knowledge of them. Jesus set the example and gave us a command to clothe, feed, and house the strangers we encounter.

Kindness inspires the recipient. It is a message that God exists and that they should feel confident in that God is real and is providing for them through you.

The difficulty to be kind will eventually resolve itself. God will get the results He designed for you to produce. He will accomplish this with any means He desires. His accomplishments and His desires require you to be kind.

When we are not kind, we are communicating two things: we think kindness costs something and we think that we are hurting someone else.

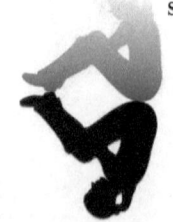

Kindness does not cost you anything. The ability to be kind is on auto-replenish from the Holy Spirit. You are not going to run out or feel empty because you are kind to others, even when they are not kind to you or you don't feel that they "deserve" kindness.

Kindness is a gift to another person. You do not know what they need and that you are in their path/presence for the reason of the gift of kindness from you.

When we are not kind, we actually hurt ourselves, because we do it out of spite for another. This is not the way of God thus we are only hurting ourselves. Consider that the Bible says what you sow you shall also reap. Translation when you are unkind, others will be unkind to you. When you are unkind, God is hurt and the ways of God are sacrificed. Kindness is not optional and repays itself.

A sweetness of temper, easy to be entreated when any have wronged us should exist in order to be kind.

Goodness

Goodness is a holistic concept inclusive of doing the right thing. Being good is a phrase first coined mostly by your parents and guardians or even your teachers. Being good is hard though, relatively unachievable. Being good requires concentration. Most of us lose our concentration trying to be good.

What is the Source of goodness? What is the definition of goodness? Who is our example of goodness? When do we become accountable for our goodness or lack thereof? Who is the recipient of our goodness? Why does the Spirit charge us to be good? Who benefits

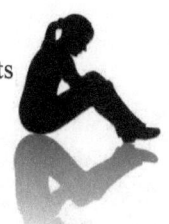

from our goodness? Are we are good? What makes it possible to be good? Conversely, what makes it impossible to be good?

The Spirit is the Source of goodness. The scripture reminds us that goodness is the fruit of the Spirit. The Spirit produces that fruit which fuels us.

Goodness is readiness to do good to all as we have opportunity. Goodness is done in spite of how we feel about doing good or about the person(s) we are commissioned to good for or with. Goodness is part of what we are called to do.

Goodness is the opposite of badness or ungoodness or anti-goodness, but more importantly anti-giving of yourself. Likewise, goodness means that we are behaving according to God's word meaning respecting authority, and taking care of God's business.

What is required for goodness to take place?

How do we influence more goodness in ourselves and others?

Faithfulness

Faithfulness is critical to have a great relationship with God. "Without faith it is impossible to please God," Hebrews 11:6. As we consider faithfulness, let us define faith. Hebrews 11:1 states that, "Faith is the substance of things hoped for and the evidence of things unseen." In short, it is believing that God is going to do and is doing what He promised in His word according to His perfect will.

Faith is a repetitive exercise of believing God anew each day for each situation, which are unique, and no situation has impact on the

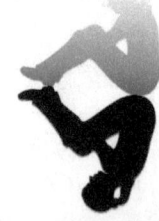

last or the next. Faith is independent of circumstance. No separate circumstances are supposed to form your faith in a fashion which is a lingering obstacle. You have let some specific instances structure your faith in a manner which will never be flexible to gain more faith. In order to have a faith which pleases God, you have to FORGET that you think that God abandoned you because your situation did not go your way! It did not go your way because your vision is limited. You knowledge is limited. There are times when God shows you how your desires would have led to your demise. This gently reminds you that your faith should grow and ultimately God was right!

    Your faith rests on the FACT that God is doing His will in each and every circumstance we experience.

    I often think that I am being faithful because I attend church, authentically worship and that I use my spiritual gifts. However, that is not the complete measure of my faith. My faith is challenged when I ask God why with an attitude that nothing should happen to me, as if I am exempt from pain, trouble, hurt. Faith means that I am committed to serving God in spite of my pain or other issues that were designed to test my relationship with God. Will I be faithful? My countenance, attitude, actions, and words should reflect my unconditional faith for God.

    Faithfulness is required to maintain a quality relationship with God. The Holy Spirit requires faith as fruit of the relationship. Faithfulness is a belief that God will do His will.

    My lifestyle should reflect my faithfulness. My faith should show my fullness in God and my walk should be a strong walk. The faith I have should be evident in my thoughts, my words, and my

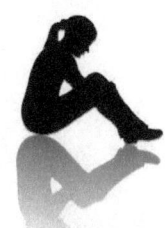

deeds. Others should know that faith is a walk of my life and a mark that I share intensely. My faith indicates I believe in the will of God.

As my faith grows stronger, my spiritual growth increases as does my relationship with God.

Gentleness

Gentleness is defined as meek and mild, lacking harshness and severity, courteous and polished. Are you gentle? I am careful not to use the same words mentioned in the verse which could be synonymous such as kindness. Gentleness is based on the nature of your spirit and is a factor of your heart.

I am not the standard gentle definition. My heart desires to show gentleness however my persona does not give off the gentleness. My presence is reported as powerful and I do not seem like I am gentle being. I know that I am working on my gentleness because I am also not the opposite of gentleness, which is violent, harshness and disdain. These definitions apply to your behavior, works and words.

Gentleness is the nature of the Spirit. Our job is to move with gentleness even when there is conflict and not bringing harm to the other parties. Gentleness is a gift to another as it is needed. Gentleness is the accurate measure of the Spirit. Most of us seek the gentle among us. When you have trouble, you naturally want some gentle words and gentle heart which is receptive to our woes. We need a place where gentleness will encourage us to keep focused on God. So are you the source of gentleness that others will seek? Can you be that person for someone else? Is gentleness a calling on our lives? I would say yes.

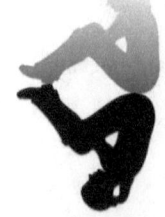

Each of us is called to do for others what we think we need and what we are asking of God.

Gentleness is contagious. Gentleness is to be shared. Gentleness is needed for life to continue. Gentleness is the basis of the hope of life. Gentleness is marked by attitude and posture.

As I grow each day, I consider how I handle others when they are placed before me. I consider who handles me gently and who I seek when I have the need to be treated gently. There are times when I fail at being gentle. One of my friends shared that he is gentle and compassionate. His compassion is an indicator of his gentleness. I had never considered that my compassion would drive my gentleness. I never paralleled the two character traits. I am a compassionate person more than I ever knew however, I question my ability to be consistently gentle.

Assume that the person you meet was sent to you by God as a test of how you will treat them. In this assumption include that he or she are in pain. Using these two details and decide that you are going to treat them well, well enough to participate in their healing. As they heal in your presence, consider how your gentleness has pleased God.

Are you gentle? Consistently? Pray to work on that trait? Remember and realize that you will receive more opportunities to be gentle to new people.

Self-control

Self-control! No one can control yourself like YOU can. SELF-CONTROL!!!

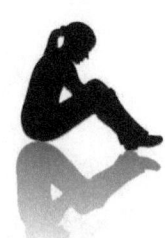

Self-control is defined by Gage as keeping yourself in check; keeping yourself within some boundaries.

Self-control is being able to keep your countenance together in a manner that will not embarrass or offend. Self-control is controlling your tongue is ALL circumstances! Do not curse. Do not "go-off." Do not lose your composure. Self-control includes being polite, knowing when to say what you think versus keeping it to yourself. How you carry yourself is that definition of self-control. How you manage your conflict is the definition of self-control.

Self-control is being faithful in your relationships and especially your marriage. Self-control is dealing with your issues in a civil manner which would not bring reproach upon you and your family.

Self-control is knowing what to wear, what is appropriate for certain occasions and events. Likewise, self-control is the definition of keeping your mouth closed based on the situation or speaking as appropriate.

Self-control is a discipline. Self-control is an example for others to follow. Self-control is a sign of maturity. This maturity is a sign of God's sovereignty on my life.

Self-control is the epitome of understanding our Christian walk. Additionally, that walk impacts others in ways that we will never imagine.

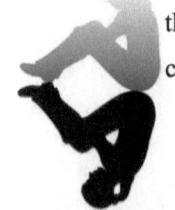

Further, the element of self-control that is key is the decision that self-control is important. The details are critical as your self-control influences others. Lack of self-control develops doubt in others about what we are supposed to do and what we are supposed to look like. Willfully breaking the covenant out the boundaries that God established is a lack of self-control.

Self-control is the respect we have for God and the reverence we have for Jesus. Self-control is what Christ uses to bring others to Christ through us. Self-control is self-accountability. Self-control means that we understand that our actions have consequences. We understand that our actions reflect on God.

Self-control is a matter of discipline and reliance on God for help in areas where self-control is lacking. Other issues which fall under the areas of self-control are issues which you would be ashamed of and would not want others to know.

Sometimes your self-control is judged by others, not by our self-perception. Others may disagree. This disagreement makes the difference.

Lifestyle

We have covered the elements of the fruit of the Spirit, which all speak to our lifestyle choices. Our lifestyle—how we live—speaks loudly about how we love God and believe His hand is on our lives.

We choose the lifestyle that we are able to show others. Who are we when no one is watching? Are we ever the purest version of ourselves? Who are we anyway? The power in that question often relies on answering who does God want us to be and who will He fashion us to become. Our answer lies in the answers we receive from Him as we spend time with Him daily. When you decide on different aspects of

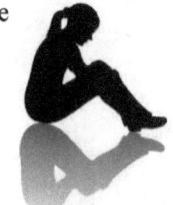

your life, you have to consider how that decision impacts your relationship with God.

I mentioned that for a few years, I did not listen to secular music. I could hear from God so much clearer than before when I was limited to gospel music not just on Sunday or during a storm.

Lifestyle defines your choice of abstinence, how much you will drink, who you will allow in your life and what other boundaries you will employ. Lifestyle considers how you handle your finances, how you will manage your education, how you manage your home, and other related choices. Lifestyle is a decision about how we will worship and serve God directly and through the lives of others. Lifestyle defines our appearance and our mannerisms and our behavior. Lifestyle dictates our friends and our friend choices.

Lifestyle separates us from the label of Christian versus the non-Christian. Yes, we sin but the willfulness and the conviction we feel when we do sin and the repentance we seek from God and Jesus is the difference.

Lifestyle is what others judge us by.

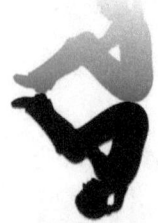

THE SPIRIT FACTOR

For the Spirit God gave us does not make us timid, but gives us power, love and self-discipline.

2 Timothy 1:7
New International Version (NIV)

For God hath not given us the Spirit of fear; but of power, and of love, and a sound mind.

2 Timothy 1:7
King James Version (KJV)

The Holy Spirit is a gift from God and Jesus for us to hold us together. The Holy Spirit molds our Spirit. The Spirit we have leads us to the best that God has for us. Likewise we need to adhere to the guidance of the Holy Spirit, who is led by God and according to God's will.

The Spirit Factor includes the factors of a healthy spirit, factors which interrupt our spirit, factors which weaken our spirit, and the factors required to build our spirit, restore or/and renew our spirit. As we cover those details of the Spirit, we will consider how to protect our spirits from the foolishness which we have previously allowed to crush, and ultimately weaken our spirits to a level which would be deemed unrecoverable.

Our spirit is the inner self which we share with others in many different manners however, the permissive sharing of our spirits with those who could hurt us is the lessons we will cover in the this chapter.

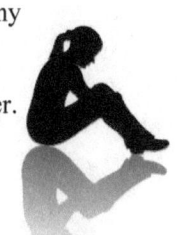

The Spirit Factor is the element that while we do not control our spirit, we control what comes into our spirit. We do not control what comes in our spirit unless we are deliberate in guarding our spirit. Our spirit warrants guarding. These are issues, materials, and people who should be denied entrance into your spirit. While we may have never considered it in this manner, we need to consider carefully who we give access to our spirits. As we consider how we got away from God from time to time, we should consider those persons, events, and materials which we have mistakenly allowed privilege to our spirit, the sacred Source of ourselves. If you could change the persons who had access to your spirit, would you? I know I would. There are persons who I should not have allowed in and in some levels I should not have entered into relationship. We don't let everyone in our spirit because they do not protect us and our spirits. They tend to take advantage of your very weaknesses and subtleties and tenderness, and your meekness. The pain was almost unrecoverable. That pain is how you know that the person should have been better monitored.

As we consider our spirit and our spirit drives our feelings, our mind, and our attitudes. With so much of what we do coming out of our spirit, why shouldn't we protect it with all that we are?

Factors for a Healthy Spirit

A healthy spirit is measured by the spiritual intake, relationship with God, recovery and resilience from issues, a consistent prayer life, and a clear understanding of pure and true love. A hearty spirit abounding in love is a healthy one as well.

A healthy spirit prevails through study, meditation and prayer. A healthy spirit requires a transparent life. Study of God's word and other related literature. The old cliché "you are what you read" is still true. What we take in with our eyes, our mouths, our minds, and our ears is what we grow with. So if we take in "junk" then we grow "junk." "So Rev. Gage does that mean that everything other than the Bible and related materials is junk?" I am glad you asked. The answer is no but too much of that without any Bible and related materials is going to produce an unhealthy spirit. Then there are materials which take your attention off of God. That is the true definition of junk.

Study of God's word is the direction of a healthy spirit. We are studying to know God and know Him better because of each encounter. We are studying to understand the events in our lives and His will in our lives. As we study God's work, His priorities are revealed and new enlightenments are exposed. Our study time offers us clarity as to what to ask from God. Study is not simply reading God's word but researching the connections of scriptures to one another and the historical attachments and implications. Study is just like observing your mate or your children or your co-workers. When you are trying to know and learn those persons, you use all available means to do so. As you do understand better that person, the love you have grows. As with God, you will experience that same growth and closeness through study.

As you grow closer to God, the more you will want to know and the closer you will want to get. Prayer is essential to the healthy spirit. Prayer is a dialogue with God. Dialogue by definition is a two-way conversation between two people who want to be in a conversation together.

YIELDED AND SUBMITTED

Prayer is a scary proposal when you consider you may have never really prayed but we seek to transform to a deeper relationship through prayer. Prayer is a reverent dialogue filled with honesty, transparency, and authenticity. God knows your heart, your mind, and the number of hairs on your head, so why do you need to pray? We pray because God seeks us through prayer. God desires us to share with Him even though He already knows. Prayer is so important to Him that He gave the Holy Spirit to intercede for us when we do not know what to pray (Romans 8:26). Prayer is so important that God gives us an Intercessor so that the fear we would have to pray would be monitored and diminished by another being.

Prayer is the intimate time with God which is not shared with others. Some aspects should be kept private. Keep in mind that God is aware of what your needs are. This is about relationship. Praise and worship requires relationship. Prayer is part of your praise and worship to God.

Meditation is the consideration of what you have read, studied, prayed and observed. Meditation is the concept of thinking over what you know. In this thought process, you should be able to reach some conclusions about direction and resolve and resolution in your life. God often speaks through meditation. Meditation also part of being still and waiting on God even though He may not utter a word. Meditation requires concentration, focus and quiet. A stillness which cannot be disturbed. Meditation is a series of quiet moments which start out small for a few minutes and overtime will evolve into 30 minutes, maybe more. The point is that you are spending quality with God.

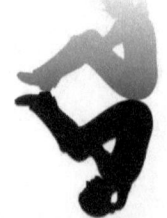

THE SPIRIT FACTOR

Leading a transparent life is a big deal and it requires all of the previously stated concepts. Gage defines transparency as sharing the real issues, the real outcomes and the real details. I have previously heard testimonies but they did not have impact on me because I could hear the gaps in the story. Those gaps indicate that REMARKABLE things happened but the testimony loses its power because the sharer does not have enough faith to share the complete testimony. What we think is that someone will judge us for what has happened to us. The problem is that what happens to us is not for us but a testimony so that others may see the end result of a storm which will offer encouragement to persevere through their own storm. Our testimonies are designed to create an understanding that "If God can do that through her then He can certainly carry my burdens and meet my needs." We have a testimony to share with others.

As I follow Christ more closely, I find out more enemies plan and plot their attacks. Unfortunately, they do not understand that when they start their attack, it has already failed. Further, when I do decide to respond to the enemy. I usually respond in such unexpected manner that the enemy is in complete confusion. My direct transparency further angers the enemy.

Finally, transparency means sharing your heart with others with the intention of invoking healing in others and remaining free of personal fear.

Factors Which Interrupt Our Spirits

By far the factors which interrupt our spirits start with sin, willful disobedience, and lack of faith. I sin. Daily. During each day, I sin. And so do you. Sin separates us from God. So God has already

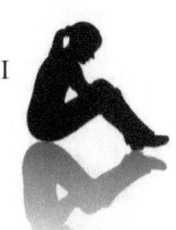

provided for us an escape from that sin. The Bible says that if we ask for forgiveness then He will forgive us in accordance to our repentance. He reconciled our sins with the death, burial, and resurrection of Jesus Christ. Sin is inevitable. Our choices make the difference when we recognize that God provides an escape when we find ourselves cornered in our own minds (1 Corinthians 10:13) and when do not choose the escape, we can seek His forgiveness.

Willful disobedience needs to be dismissed. I struggle daily with willful disobedience. I struggle daily with willful disobedience. It covers something as small as eating more than you should to pre-marital sex or adultery. It is a matter of discipline. Sometimes I lack discipline and I sin willfully. I have to still repent. I also ask for better assistance for escape and will power to do what will please God. I am reminded of a scripture which is the ultimate in discipleship, Luke 9:23: "Then He said to them all: "Whoever wants to be my disciple must deny themselves and take up their cross and follow Me."" God wants us to understand that our personal cravings and selfishness need to be dismissed so that Christ can be glorified, magnified and kept first.

Lack of faith is highly offensive to God. Imagine that we did not create ourselves yet we DOUBT, QUESTION, IGNORE and DISOBEY the ONE who did. Hebrews 11:6 reads: "Without faith it is impossible to please God." So faith is important to you spirit and your relationship with God. Faith is evident in our words and deeds. There is actual evidence which communicates to God and shares it with others.

Factors Which Weaken Our Spirit

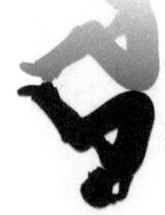

If study, prayer, and meditation strengthens your spirit, then obviously incomplete, improper or inconsistent study, prayer and meditation weakens your spirit. I am sure that I could create a formula that speaks to how much study, prayer and meditation you should take in based on how much you take in which is designed to cause you trouble, pain and other issues. I doubt I need to do that because by virtue of common sense, you know that you have to take more in good than bad so that you can maintain a healthy margin for a healthy spirit.

After that works for you, consider those things that facilitate your bad attitude, your frowns, your dismal disposition, your tenacious tone, your poor posture and challenged mental capacity. The factors which contribute to the weakened spirit include the male companion, the family, the career and the social/emotional considerations. As you pour over these aspects, consider what those issues are and how can they can be solved so that they can be removed from the equation.

Depression is medically real and the contributing factors are a reality. We cannot avoid the medical issues created by stress, anxiety and worry. The result is depression and emotional poverty. These actual medical issues require God, maybe medication and a HUGE decision to get past that situation. These are based on situations and circumstances. This is not who you are and does not define who you will be.

Addictions are a factor as well. Food. Sex. Social Networking. Shopping. Smoking. Drugs. Alcohol. Television. Entertainment. Work. Relationships. Reading. Activities which require you to take time away from God. Things that make you hide from God. Addictions are hard to admit, reconcile, and redirect that energy toward a better place.

Addictions are hard on your loved ones. They see you try to hide the addiction but it is difficult to do so with the level that you were hoping. Understand that addictions can be healed and your family will love you through that healing. Jesus recalls that you need to confess your addiction(s), seek healing and COMMIT to that recovery. The word of God says that "not by might or power but by the Spirit of God (Zechariah 4:6)."

I dated a man with an addiction to pornography. When I found out about it, I asked him about it. He denied it. I pleaded with him about helping him. I had promised to love him unconditionally through his eventual healing. The problem is that he shut me out. He denied. He lied. He failed to acknowledge the value of what I presented. I left because that relationship was no longer healthy for my spirit. Keep in mind unconditional love requires two people—both of whom recognize God as Lord. He placed his addiction before God and me. God has to do that work.

Maybe you are the addict. Seek help and do not reject those who love you as you heal.

Maybe you are the outsider. Pray. Seek God's face and guidance during this time. Your loved ones need you and NOT your judgment. FAST on their behalf. Love them through their storm. Always keep in mind that you would want and frankly expect that UNCONDITIONAL LOVE. Treat them the way you would have them treat you.

Other factors such as depression, bulimia, and other issues which develop into medical issues. All of which require our love. John 13:34-35 reads [34] "A new command I give you: Love one another. As I have loved you, so you must love one another. [35] By this everyone will know that you are my disciples, if you love one another."

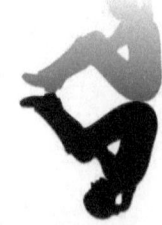

This commandment is an expression of Jesus' love for us and how we should love each other. Authentic love has the power to restore your spirit.

Factors Which Rebuild Our Spirit

Pray.

Study.

Meditate.

Fast.

Love.

Share.

Confess.

Authenticity.

Genuineness.

Of all of those factors, the one aspect we have not covered is being true to oneself. Stop being FAKE! First with yourself, then with others. It takes great courage to be the real you. For most of us, we do not even know who WE are. Being real is definitely difficult when we do not know who that is. The mirror is a great starting place. Look at yourself in the mirror until you start to appreciate who are staring at and investigating.

Love yourself by FORGIVING yourself. Whatever you have done and endured is over and now you have to step into your life. Dive

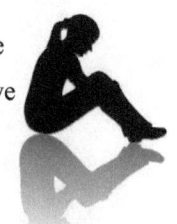

in completely. AUTHENTICALLY. That means that you seek the truth within yourself. That means that you seek the truth within yourself. That means that you consider your past as your past and move on from there.

Stand firm in what you do know about yourself. Realize that you need to understand that God loves you regardless of what that past is. Your past could be compared to that of Saul who was later converted to Paul. Saul had spoken out against Jesus in a lot of audiences. Acts 9 shares his story. God has designed you for His purposes and He will insure that your life will look like what He designed.

Stop the negative self-talk! Negativity cannot stay inside your heart. Your heart and spirit are in communion with one another. Negativity cannot exist and those entities remain healthy.

"There Ain't No Quit In Me!" You have to decide to be focused on God and not let other "stuff" interfere with what God wants you to do. I personally cannot afford to consider quitting. God put me here to work for HIM. Everything I do needs to bring Him glory. If I quit, then my work cannot be done. If I quit, then God is not glorified as He initially designed. If I quit, then those who watch me and know me may abandon hope, and then they may quit as well. I have personally experienced some things that should have shaken my faith, could have interrupted my relationship with God, and would have made me uncertain of my future. God has not left me and has kept me close to Him, continuing to protect me and love me and provide for me.

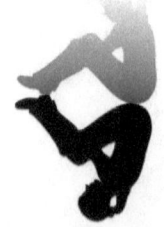

How Do I Know that I Need to Rebuild and Replenish My Spirit

I did a radio show where I shared how you know that you are not holding on to old stuff. You need to rebuild on a regular basis. When you build your spirit, study, reading, prayer, and meditation are essential. This rebuilding is evident through your words, deeds, thoughts, and eyes. Eyes? Yes, your eyes share your issue. Your eyes speak to your situation. When you are sad, your eyes show it. When you are excited, your eyes show it. There are depths to your eyes which communicates volumes about how are doing internally. How you are feeling, which is the output of your spirit, is reflected through your eyes, your body language, your tone, and your words. And your image.

Your body language is a clear indication that you need to build your spirit. If you are stiff and hard toward others, then you are functioning with a weak spirit. Your body language communicates with others that you are approachable and open to sharing and being personable. Your image is important. How you feel should only be reflected if you feel great! With that said, understand that you <u>always</u> need to look like you feel great! NO EXCUSES!!! If you don't feel like looking great, STAY HOME!!! When people see you, they judge you! They may not say anything when you look bad, but they are judging you and wondering about your situation.

When we look great, we receive compliments. Those compliments lift our spirits. We need that lift no matter your situation. When you have sacrificed your image because you don't feel like it, they further unseat your spirit through their comments and judgment.

Your words signify your spiritual bankruptcy. When your words are rough, harsh, rude, ugly, and hurting others, you are

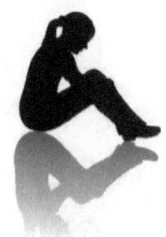

spiritually in the negative. Spiritual bankruptcy can be recovered through prayer, study, meditation, fasting, healing and love of God because He loved you first. He loves and He loved you first. Your words will be peaceful, discreet, loving, gracious, edifying, building, forgiving, and purposed with wisdom. Your words should build up others. You should be sought for wisdom through your words and thoughts. Your words should comfort and not diminish others. Your words should settle and not agitate or aggravate. Your words can cause death or create life and the choice is yours of which you do in the lives of others. Your words are an indicator of where you are.

Take a break. Take a break for yourself. Replenish with time spent alone with God: study, meditate, read and pray. Schedule your breaks so that you do not have arrive at spiritual bankruptcy. You are better able to rebuild with some wellness than from nothing—bankruptcy.

Power, Love and Self-Discipline Not Fear

Finally to the scripture, 2 Timothy 1:7, your spirit was built for power, love, and self-discipline not fear. God gave us power, love, and self-discipline. Because of the Source, we should never be empty. No such bankruptcy should ever exist. Fear comes from many sources but not from God. Actually, your fear offends God. Fear says to God that whatever you are afraid of is bigger than God. It means that you do not trust God with that situation. Fear and power, love and self-discipline cannot co-exist. God can handle your whole situation. ALL of it.

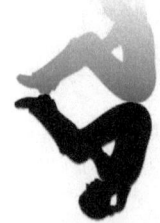

Power, love and self-discipline exist so that we can serve God completely.

When we discussed the need to rebuild of your spirit on a regular basis so that you can purge that negativity, this is critical to maintain the health of the power, love, and self-discipline that God offers. Each of us needs to do it. Meditation, vacations, and retreats are important for this as well as honestly addressing your fears. Ask God for help navigating your fears—those details of your life that you do not want to deal with. Once you address those things, you have a lighter spirit.

Self-discipline is given by God. You <u>can</u> say NO. You can avoid the temptation. You can change your attitude, your actions, and your outlook. All with that God already gave you.

I know that some of us need medications for some specific issues, however, all of us do not have that need. For those of us who do not have a medical need, we have an excuse! Ouch! I know. We are using an excuse to behave badly, sin purposely and live foolishly. This cannot any longer be acceptable. Stop doing and stop accepting it from those around you.

Find ways to obey more and sin less. God is counting on our best behavior. Self-discipline and the lack thereof can negatively affect your love and power. Fear stifles our abilities and our influence. As we develop our spirits and further develop our spirits to share our spirit with others, we need to consider that we will have to change.

The challenge is to recognize the parts of power, love, and self-discipline which needs to be sharpened so that we can know where our best details are so that it is easier to develop the stuff which needs help.

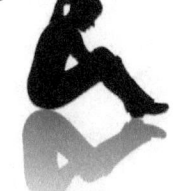

YIELDED AND SUBMITTED

When I get "scared," I recall this scripture. When I hear others communicate fear, I share this scripture.

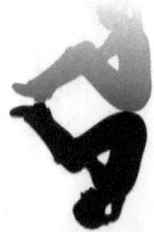

A WOMAN'S JOURNEY FOR A LIFE DEDICATED TO GOD

THE SELF-ESTEEM FACTOR

I praise You because I am fearfully and wonderfully made; Your works are wonderful and I know that full well.

Psalm 139:14 (NIV)

Our self-esteem is quite delicate. One word, one gesture, one action can change the substance and concept of the self-esteem of a person. Our self-esteem is the report card of who we have become because of our experiences and persons who influence our lives and the words they use. Our self-esteem drives our decisions and choices. When I make a poorly researched choice, I start with my self-esteem: did my personal deficit make this happen? Our self-esteem is critical to how we relate to others. Self-esteem is the outcome of your education, experiences, and most importantly, how you were made to feel about those experiences.

Self-esteem is shaped by love, forgiveness, self-doubt, faith, belief, stress, struggles, fear and peace. When I consider my own self-esteem, there are areas which I need some support and some sustaining. Women, you are to protect your self-esteem. Your self-esteem is evidence of your life. The factors are "daddy," "mommy," background, your image and your relationships.

Our self-esteem is formed by all of the persons we have close relationships with. Self-esteem is internal yet based on the external influences, some of which we are unaware of its potential harm.

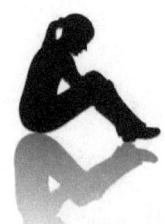

Beauty is defined as an internal and external match of looks, charm, presence and mental prowess. You are beautiful. You control that beauty by what you consume in your spiritual food, mental food, physical food, and your outward appearance. Your self-esteem is aligned with that beauty until you give away the controls.

As a little girl, I thought the world revolved around me and maybe you thought the same. The world revolved around me because I am smart and pretty and have nice clothes and my daddy confirmed that information on a regular basis. As a little girl, we do not immediately understand or experience hurt. But then it happens: DIVORCE. The affirmation stops. The words become negative—you are just like your father. My mother's bitterness became my reality.

As I become a young lady, she still had not recovered. She is not only bitter, now she is jealous of her own child. The only child that has not embarrassed her and that has been successful.

This is not a special or unique story. It is not even scary or ugly. It is real. Like so many of your stories and that of your friends and family, these events affected our self-esteem. The next step is the critical piece: YOU MAKE A CHOICE. You keep it or resign from it. I decided early, about age 16, that my life would not be governed by my family's foolishness.

Our Choices

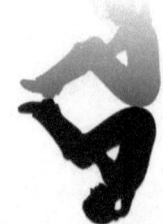

The relationships we keep and nurture are ones which should nurture and affirm us. No, they are not going to co-sign on your foolishness. They are going to love you and hold you accountable.

They are going to encourage you and share with you. They are going to believe in you and criticize you. They are going to see you for the potential you have. They are going to stop you from putting yourself in harm's way and putting yourself down. They are going to create you a safe place for you to speak about your needs and dreams and fears. They are going to protect you from those who want to hurt you.

These are the standards by which we measure and manage these relationships. Keep in mind you govern whether or not people have access to you and your stuff. Keep in mind you can offer access or limit that access or reverse that access at any time. You have to be honest with yourself about why people are really in your life. Act accordingly for the health of your self-esteem. The wrong person can bring continued havoc in your life. You already know this but you are not great at moving them to the outer relationship marker. Let's work on that.

Our Actions

Our personal actions and words need to match. People measure you by your words and actions matching. This is the answer to 'why don't people take me seriously.' Do you do what you say you are going to do. Your 'no' needs to mean 'no.' Likewise, your 'yes' needs to mean 'yes.' Maintain and advertise your standards. Be careful about who you let in. If you are more careful then you do not reject so many people. Damage control and clean-up would not be so hard.

Our Decisions

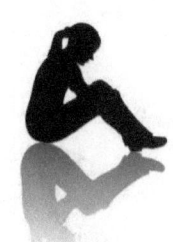

Our decisions are based on how we feel about ourselves. You have let your "best friend" talk down to you because you did not believe in yourself. You have selected the wrong men because you do not think you deserve better. You do not pursue your dreams because someone told you that you were never going to be anybody.

You agreed with them because your self-esteem has been damaged.

Our Changes

Decide to understand who God made you to be. Your self-esteem, self-value, and self-worth was made by God. Any changes which have been made to your self-esteem were done by you and those you allow access. If only He could reset you to His factory settings, but that is not possible. So since we cannot be reset to the original settings, we have to return to the original directions and to the Author and Creator.

Our scripture Psalm 139:14 "I praise You because I am fearfully and wonderfully made; Your works are wonderful and I know that full well."

Consider if you believed that you are fearfully and wonderfully made, how would you behave? I imagine the confidence that God really gave you to do His will. Remember that we are made in His image and all that that includes. How would we behave differently if we believed we were wonderful? Not a prideful wonderful but a wonderful which keeps us from doubting the God who created us using His image as the pattern to create me, developed with carefully

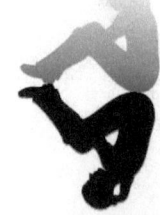

constructed places with dates and times He has carefully planned so that I can be the daughter He deserves.

Our fragmented and fragile self-esteem interrupts our relationship with God. The self-esteem we are supposed to have is one that openly praises God and seeking Him is priority. How do we start to reflect the intended factory settings? How do we return to a self-esteem which pleases God? How do we reach a place where we stop grieving God because we do not behave?

Our first change is an understanding that the scripture is for us. God made us and He made us durable and resilient. The events, activities and people that happen to us are to build character and emotional muscle and to remind us of why we have a God.

Our second change is to decide to believe His words—all of them. Psalm 139:14. Ephesians 2:8-10. Proverbs 31:10-31. Genesis 1:26-27. Matthew 22:37. Jeremiah 29:11. Matthew 10:30-31. Jeremiah 1:5. God's words are true about you. All of them!

Our third change is to disregard, dismiss, discount, disengage, all, ALL of the negative words and thoughts and comments and actions which tug and eat and disturb that very essence of who you are and which are reflected in your damaged self-esteem. These are very things that have caused your self-esteem to weary, weaken, wither, waiver and wrinkle. These events, actions, activities and actors are designed to drive you back to God and cause a refreshing, realignment and a reinvestment in your relationship with God.

So the fourth change is to pray for reconciliation, restoration, and reclamation with regards to our self-esteem and ultimately to God Himself. God can heal us from our issues as well as deliver us into a place when we can share our testimonies with others. This requires you to forgive yourself for whatever you have been holding over your own head. God forgives and heals. The question is can you allow it and accept it. Live with it. And move forward.

So the fifth change would be reconstructing how we make decisions and how we respond to others. Understand by this I mean rejecting our old behavior and considering how to select the better choice. Stop rationalizing our own foolishness because of our desperation. Or whatever excuse has previously brought us comfort. We have affairs because of our low self-esteem. We let him physically and emotionally abuse us because of low self-esteem. We are overweight because of low self-esteem. We avoid our own success because of low self-esteem. We stay in our own rut because of that low self-esteem. God can see to it that we overcome these obstacles and issues. YES, GOD CAN and WILL!

Your healthy self-esteem requires God's intervention. Please seek Him.

Our Resolve

In 1998, I decided to be abstinent. I made the decision at a youth conference, True Love Waits, with 25 young people and 3 other youth workers. I was going to say no to premarital sex. I asked God to help me; to relieve me of the desire and prepare me for my mate.

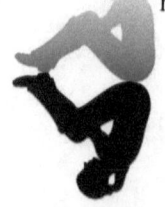

Through this commitment to abstinence, I learned that my self-esteem was attached to my vagina. I believed that when he slept with me that sex validated who I was. I was totally transformed by this commitment. I learned that if I wanted a man to know me then sex need to be omitted. As I learned this valuable lesson, I had to be truly transparent. I met a man and as I introduced myself I would include that I was abstinent. MANY walked away immediately. SOME held a conversation. A FEW wanted to go on a date. So the bottom line was that I had to learn my worth was between my ears, in the confines of my heart and deep within my spirit, not in my physical intimacy. When I learned this, I was able to walk away from unhealthy relationships, identify unhealthy relationships and wait.

There are people who are mean and that poor behavior and attitude is a reflection of low self-esteem. The resolve is that we recognize it, give it over to God, and watch God work.

A healthy self-esteem allows us to be completely yielded and submitted to God the way God designed.

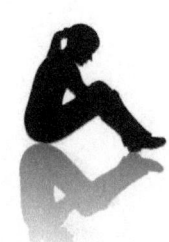

YIELDED AND SUBMITTED

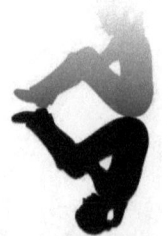

Conclusion

Yielded and Submitted: A Woman's Journey for a Life Dedicated to God has been my testimony. I hope that you have grown as much as I have. I consider this a complete blessing to have written this book where you can grow closer to God through my transparency. I certainly think that this was an interesting project assigned to me by God. As I considered what He had me to write, I certainly thought that it would be hard for me to share but God allowed me to give you what He had done it my life so that you could grow.

God gives through people so that they can give to others. May God bless you as you journey back to God. He's waiting for you to return to the complete comfort of His arms and so you can better hear His voice. God considers you His best work.

Who will share this information or revelation with?

What do you think I need to be sure to avoid as a woman?

How has this helped you grow?

What do you do now:

> Goals?
>
> Changes?
>
> Prayer Closet?
>
> Do you love with your whole heart?

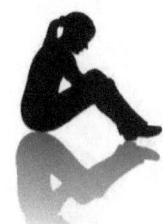

Please share your testimonies and prayers; prayer requests and praise reports at onediagage@onediagage.com. I look forward to hearing from you.

The Benediction

[24] The LORD bless you and keep you;
[25] the LORD make His face shine on you and be gracious to you;
[26] the LORD turn his face toward you and give you peace."

Numbers 6:24-26 (NIV)

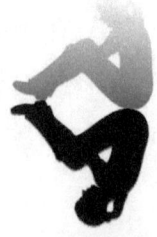

RESOURCES

The Scriptures

What God Says About His Word

"All Scripture is God-breathed and is useful for teaching, rebuking, correcting and training in righteousness, so that the man of God may be thoroughly equipped for every good work." 2 Timothy 3:16-17

"In the beginning was the Word, and the Word was with God, and the Word was God. He was with God in the beginning." John 1:1-2

Why Memorize Scriptures

"I have hidden Your word in my heart that I might not sin against You." Psalm 119:11

"Let the word of Christ dwell in you richly as you teach and admonish one another with all wisdom, and as you sing psalms, hymns and spiritual songs with gratitude in your hearts to God." Colossians 3:16

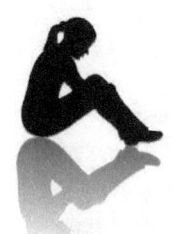

My Favorite Scriptures

Numbers 6:24-26

²⁴ The LORD bless you and keep you;
²⁵ the LORD make his face shine on you and be gracious to you;
²⁶ the LORD turn his face toward you and give you peace."

Jeremiah 1:5

⁵ "Before I formed you in the womb I knew you, before you were born I set you apart; I appointed you as a prophet to the nations."

Jeremiah 29:11

¹¹ For I know the plans I have for you," declares the LORD, "plans to prosper you and not to harm you, plans to give you hope and a future.

Psalm 1

¹ Blessed is the one
who does not walk in step with the wicked
or stand in the way that sinners take
or sit in the company of mockers,
² but whose delight is in the law of the LORD,
and who meditates on his law day and night.
³ That person is like a tree planted by streams of water,
which yields its fruit in season
and whose leaf does not wither—
whatever they do prospers.

⁴ Not so the wicked!
They are like chaff
that the wind blows away.

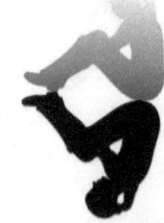

⁵ Therefore the wicked will not stand in the judgment,
nor sinners in the assembly of the righteous.

⁶ For the LORD watches over the way of the righteous,
but the way of the wicked leads to destruction.

Psalm 8

¹ LORD, our Lord,
how majestic is your name in all the earth!

You have set your glory
in the heavens.
² Through the praise of children and infants
you have established a stronghold against your enemies,
to silence the foe and the avenger.
³ When I consider your heavens,
the work of your fingers,
the moon and the stars,
which you have set in place,
⁴ what is mankind that you are mindful of them,
human beings that you care for them?[c]

⁵ You have made them[d] a little lower than the angels[e]
and crowned them[f] with glory and honor.
⁶ You made them rulers over the works of your hands;
you put everything under their[g] feet:
⁷ all flocks and herds,
and the animals of the wild,
⁸ the birds in the sky,
and the fish in the sea,
all that swim the paths of the seas.

⁹ LORD, our Lord,
how majestic is your name in all the earth!

Psalm 19:14

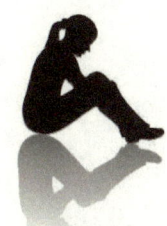

YIELDED AND SUBMITTED

¹⁴ May these words of my mouth and this meditation of my heart be pleasing in your sight, LORD, my Rock and my Redeemer.

Psalm 23 (KJV)

¹The LORD is my shepherd; I shall not want.

²He maketh me to lie down in green pastures: he leadeth me beside the still waters.

³He restoreth my soul: he leadeth me in the paths of righteousness for his name's sake.

⁴Yea, though I walk through the valley of the shadow of death, I will fear no evil: for thou art with me; thy rod and thy staff they comfort me.

⁵Thou preparest a table before me in the presence of mine enemies: thou anointest my head with oil; my cup runneth over.

⁶Surely goodness and mercy shall follow me all the days of my life: and I will dwell in the house of the LORD forever.

Psalm 46:1

¹ God is our refuge and strength,
an ever-present help in trouble.

Psalm 46:10

¹⁰ "Be still, and know that I am God;
I will be exalted among the nations,
I will be exalted in the earth."

Psalm 100

¹ Shout for joy to the LORD, all the earth.
² Worship the LORD with gladness;

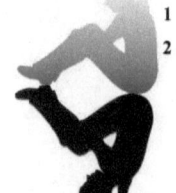

come before him with joyful songs.
³ Know that the LORD is God.
It is he who made us, and we are his[a];
we are his people, the sheep of his pasture.

⁴ Enter his gates with thanksgiving
and his courts with praise;
give thanks to him and praise his name.
⁵ For the LORD is good and his love endures forever;
his faithfulness continues through all generations.

Psalm 119:11

¹¹ I have hidden your word in my heart that I might not sin against you.

Psalm 139:14

¹⁴ I praise you because I am fearfully and wonderfully made; your works are wonderful, I know that full well.

Proverbs 3:5-6

⁵ Trust in the LORD with all your heart and lean not on your own understanding;
⁶ in all your ways acknowledge him, and he will make your paths straight.

Proverbs 23:7 (KJV)

⁷For as he thinketh in his heart, so is he: Eat and drink, saith he to thee; but his heart is not with thee.

Habakkuk 2:2

² Then the LORD replied:

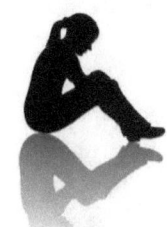

"Write down the revelation
and make it plain on tablets
so that a herald[a] may run with it.

Matthew 11:28, 30

[28] "Come to me, all you who are weary and heavy-ladened, and I will give you rest.

[30] For my yoke is easy and my burden is light."

Matthew 14:31

[31] Immediately Jesus reached out his hand and caught him. "You of little faith," he said, "why did you doubt?"

Matthew 22:37

[37] Jesus replied: "'Love the Lord your God with all your heart and with all your soul and with all your mind.

Matthew 28:19-20

[19] Therefore go and make disciples of all nations, baptizing them in[a] the name of the Father and of the Son and of the Holy Spirit, [20] and teaching them to obey everything I have commanded you. And surely I am with you always, to the very end of the age."

Luke 9:23-24

[23] Then he said to them all: "If anyone would come after me, he must deny himself and take up his cross daily and follow me. [24] For whoever wants to save his life will lose it, but whoever loses his life for me will save it.

Luke 23:34

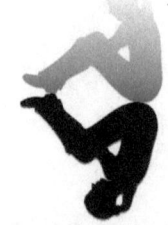

[34] Jesus said, "Father, forgive them, for they do not know what they are doing."[a] And they divided up his clothes by casting lots.

John 1:1-2

[1] In the beginning was the Word, and the Word was with God, and the Word was God. [2] He was with God in the beginning.

John 3:16

[16] "For God so loved the world that he gave his one and only Son,[a] that whoever believes in him shall not perish but have eternal life.

John 3:30

[30] He must become greater; I must become less.

John 11:35

[35] Jesus wept.

Romans 8:26

[26] In the same way, the Spirit helps us in our weakness. We do not know what we ought to pray for, but the Spirit himself intercedes for us with groans that words cannot express.

1 Corinthians 10:13

[13] No temptation has seized you except what is common to man. And God is faithful; he will not let you be tempted beyond what you can bear. But when you are tempted, he will also provide a way out so that you can stand up under it.

Galatians 5:22-23

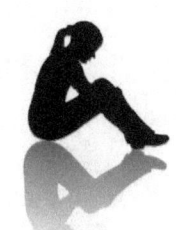

²² But the fruit of the Spirit is love, joy, peace, patience, kindness, goodness, faithfulness, ²³ gentleness and self-control. Against such things there is no law.

Ephesians 3:14-21

¹⁴ For this reason I kneel before the Father, ¹⁵ from whom his whole family[a] in heaven and on earth derives its name. ¹⁶ I pray that out of his glorious riches he may strengthen you with power through his Spirit in your inner being, ¹⁷ so that Christ may dwell in your hearts through faith. And I pray that you, being rooted and established in love, ¹⁸ may have power, together with all the saints, to grasp how wide and long and high and deep is the love of Christ, ¹⁹ and to know this love that surpasses knowledge—that you may be filled to the measure of all the fullness of God.

²⁰ Now to him who is able to do immeasurably more than all we ask or imagine, according to his power that is at work within us, ²¹ to him be glory in the church and in Christ Jesus throughout all generations, for ever and ever! Amen.

Ephesians 4:26-27

²⁶ "In your anger do not sin": Do not let the sun go down while you are still angry, ²⁷ and do not give the devil a foothold.

Ephesians 4:32

³² Be kind and compassionate to one another, forgiving each other, just as in Christ God forgave you.

Philippians 4:7

⁷ And the peace of God, which transcends all understanding, will guard your hearts and your minds in Christ Jesus.

Philippians 4:13-17

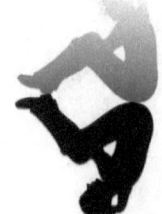

¹³ I can do everything through him who gives me strength.

¹⁴ Yet it was good of you to share in my troubles. ¹⁵ Moreover, as you Philippians know, in the early days of your acquaintance with the gospel, when I set out from Macedonia, not one church shared with me in the matter of giving and receiving, except you only; ¹⁶ for even when I was in Thessalonica, you sent me aid again and again when I was in need. ¹⁷ Not that I am looking for a gift, but I am looking for what may be credited to your account.

Colossians 3:23

²³ Whatever you do, work at it with all your heart, as working for the Lord, not for men,

1 Thessalonians 5:17

¹⁷ pray continually;

Hebrews 11:6

⁶ And without faith it is impossible to please God, because anyone who comes to him must believe that he exists and that he rewards those who earnestly seek him.

Hebrews 13:5b

⁵ Keep your lives free from the love of money and be content with what you have, because God has said,

"Never will I leave you;
never will I forsake you."

James 1:2-5

² Consider it pure joy, my brothers, whenever you face trials of many kinds, ³ because you know that the testing of your faith

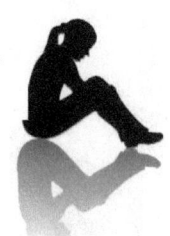

develops perseverance. ⁴ Perseverance must finish its work so that you may be mature and complete, not lacking anything. ⁵ If any of you lacks wisdom, he should ask God, who gives generously to all without finding fault, and it will be given to him.

Jude 24

²⁴Now unto him that is able to keep you from falling, and to present you faultless before the presence of his glory with exceeding joy,

Revelation 3:16

¹⁶ So, because you are lukewarm—neither hot nor cold—I am about to spit you out of my mouth.

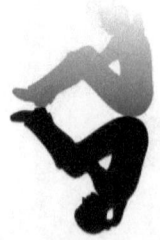

A WOMAN'S JOURNEY FOR A LIFE DEDICATED TO GOD

THE BOOKS

The Power of the Praying Parent by Stormie Omartian

The Power of the Praying Wife by Stormie Omartian

The Power of the Praying Husband by Stormie Omartian

The Power of Praying Together by Stormie Omartian

A Woman After God's Own Heart by Elizabeth George

The Five Love Languages by Dr. Gary Chapman

Friends, Lovers and Soul Mates by Drs. Darlene & Derek Hopson

My Utmost for His Highest by Oswald Chambers

God Chasers by Tommy Tenney

God Catchers by Tommy Tenney

As We Grow Together Daily Devotional for Expectant Couples by Onedia N. Gage

As We Grow Together Prayer Journal for Expectant Couples by Onedia N. Gage

The Blue Print: Poetry for the Soul by Onedia N. Gage

In Purple Ink: Poetry for the Spirit by Onedia N. Gage

Living An Authentic Life by Onedia N. Gage

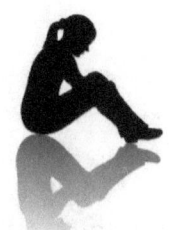

YIELDED AND SUBMITTED

On This Journey Daily Devotional for Young People by Onedia N. Gage

On This Journey Prayer Journal for Young People by Onedia N. Gage

Promises, Promises by Onedia N. Gage

Kingdom Woman by Tony Evans

Kingdom Man by Tony Evans

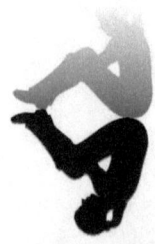

A WOMAN'S JOURNEY FOR A LIFE DEDICATED TO GOD

STUDY RESOURCES

Experiencing God

Disciple's Prayer Life

The Beloved Disciple: A Study of John

Ephesians

David: Seeking a Heart Like His

MasterLife

Abide in Christ

Fellowship with Believers

Live in the Word

Minister to Others

Pray in Faith

Witness to the World

Living God's Word

Hearing God's Voice

When God Speaks

In My Father's House

Esther

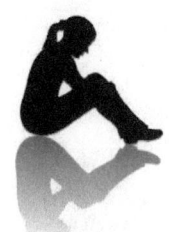

YIELDED AND SUBMITTED

WEBSITES

www.onediagage.com

www.lifeway.com

www.stormieomartian.com

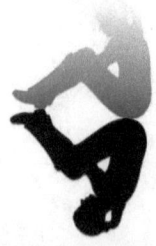

ACKNOWLEDGMENTS

God, thank You for Your plans for me. Thank You for *Yielded and Submitted: A Woman's Journey for a Life Dedicated to God* and choosing me to complete Your project. I just want to please You. Thank You for continuing to anoint me and to invest in me and my gifts, which keep surprising me. Thank You for loving and forgiving me.

Hillary and Nehemiah, thank you for supporting me and my endeavors. Thank you for loving me, especially when I do nothing without a pen and a clipboard, thank you for enduring my late nights, your ideas, the sounding board, the love and the support. Thank you for celebrating our legacy.

To my reading team: Rev. A. Canady, Minister M. Fowler, Minister D. Kennebrew and Mr. G. Wyche, Jr. Thanks for the feedback and the discussions. The bantering has grown me and my writing. Your subjectivity and objectivity shed light on my project.

To my prayer partners and to my accountability partners, thank you for the long talks and the powerful prayers and the encouragement.

To the women who this will reach and empower and touch and affect, may these words empower you and help you fervently seek God and reach some resolve. May you be inspired to achieve your goals and dreams. May you enhance your relationship with God so that your other relationships will also improve. May you enhance your self-esteem through prayer and studying. May you have courage and peace. Share love the best you can until you can share love without reservation.

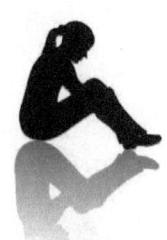

YIELDED AND SUBMITTED

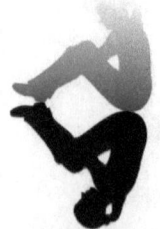

Minister Onedia N. Gage wants women to have the help she wanted and needed as she seeks a stronger relationship with God. She always seeks God for leadership, guidance, and comfort.

Take her advice and testimony seriously. Her experience is invaluable. Please use this to reach God. Yielding and Submitting is worth it—on every level.

Please feel free to contact her at www.onediagage.com and onediagage@onediagage.com. Follow her on twitter.com @onediangage.

www.ingramcontent.com/pod-product-compliance
Lightning Source LLC
Chambersburg PA
CBHW020938180426
43194CB00038B/373